Age Busters

Age Busters

Simple Steps to Enhance Your Life and Beat Stress

Charles A. Salter

and

Carlota de Lerma Salter

CITADEL PRESS
Kensington Publishing Corp.
www.kensingtonbooks.com

First printing: January 2002

10 9 8 7 6 5 4 3 2 1

Printed in the United States of America

Library of Congress Control Number: 2001092402

ISBN 0-8065-2234-8

We dedicate this book to our son Brian and his wife Claudia, our elder daughter Valerie and her fiancé Ray, and our younger daughter Carolyn. You have always been a great joy to us. Thank you for your prayers, love, and encouragement.

CONTENTS

PART III: PROTECT YOUR BODY

PART IV: BUILD BETTER HABITS

PART V: WORK TOWARD DELIGHTFUL RELATIONSHIPS

PART VI: ENHANCE EMOTIONAL HEALTH

ACKNOWLEDGMENTS

The authors would like to thank Ms. Carrie Cantor for helping to develop the original concept for this book; Mr. Robert Shuman for helping to shape its final form; and Mr. Jack Alspaugh for providing the artwork in chapter 1 on stretching.

We would also like to thank Drs. Luis and Carlota de Lerma for providing their medical expertise, as well as their proofreading and editing skills. We would also like to thank our friends Henry and Debbie Erbes for their support and assistance in gathering research material. Finally, we would like to express our gratitude to Carolyn Salter for her assistance with the editing process and for giving up so much of her time and activities so we could meet our deadlines.

INTRODUCTION

"**F**ollow this simple plan for minutes a day, prevent all disease, and live a hundred-plus years in perfect health!" Blah, blah, blah . . .

Sounds great, doesn't it? But that's just make-believe. No book you read, no pill you buy, no potion you take can turn you into a permanent twenty-two-year-old. So let's forget about happy fantasy and get real.

What *is* possible?

How about reversing many of the signs of aging, such as clogged arteries, bloated bellies, and gasping for breath after climbing a flight of stairs? How about slowing down the inevitable aging process, so that when you're really sixty you have the body and performance and well-being of a fifty-year-old—or even a forty-five-year-old? How about extending the life span beyond the average and—better than that—making those extra years healthier and happier right up until near the end?

Wonderful benefits like these, based on the newest findings in medicine, nutrition, and psychology, are realistic. This book provides a blueprint to a healthier you, to a happier future.

Is this all just armchair theorizing? No. Take Charles's mother, for instance, who follows many (but not all yet) of the principles outlined in this book. As of this writing, she is seventy-nine years old and still works. One of her jobs is caring for fellow senior citizens who are confined to their own homes. Some of them are younger than she is, yet they're no longer able to manage life alone, while she's fully capable of taking care of herself, driving to work, and caring for others. In which condition do you want to be at seventy-nine? Would you like to slow your biological clock, bust the many signs of age, and restore many of the qualities of your youth?

About the Authors

Charles holds five earned university degrees, including two doctorates—a B.S. from Tulane University, an M.A. and Ph.D. in psychology from the University of Pennsylvania, and an M.S. in general nutrition and a doctor of science (S.D.) in neurobehavioral nutrition from Harvard University. He holds two state licenses, one in each of the fields of psychology and nutrition. He has published a dozen books, mostly in the areas of food, nutrition, and health, and hundreds of articles in many fields of science and medicine. He has taught at several colleges and universities, including Harvard. Currently, he travels the world teaching special seminars to doctors, nurses, and other medical professionals at major hospitals. In recent years, he has given such medical lectures throughout the United States, including Alaska and Hawaii; in Europe; in the Middle East (Bahrain); in the Far East (mainland Japan, Okinawa, South Korea); and in Australia.

His coauthor and wife is Carlota. She holds two university degrees, including a master's degree in social gerontology—the psychology, sociology, and biology of aging. She was one of the first students in the country to earn an interdisciplinary degree in this field. She has worked as a social gerontologist and certified therapeutic recreational specialist (C.T.R.S.) in geriatric centers, state hospitals, nursing homes, and in-home health care. Together, Charles and Carlota have conducted research, published articles, and given oral presentations in the field of aging for more than twenty-five years.

About This Book

This book gives you fifty-two ways to enhance every aspect of your life through such things as better health care, exercise, nutrition, psychology, and relationships. Why fifty-two? One for each week of the year. You'll no doubt want to read the whole book straight through right away. But it's hard to make a large number of life changes all at once. Therefore, we recommend that you go back and put into practice what you have learned—but gradually. You could implement a dozen or more ideas at once, if you wish. But one convenient plan suggests you spend a week on each chapter, fully implementing every option and integrating each with all the material from previous chapters. That way, in one year you could completely revolutionize every facet of your life and maximize your potential for a long and healthy life span.

The fifty-two chapters in this book are organized into several fundamental categories. First, we'll examine various aspects of exercise to get you started off right. In later sections, we'll deal with food, diet, and nutrition; medical and safety issues; building better habits; enhancing your relationships; and finally, maximizing emotional health for a long and happy life.

One caution: please consult your physician before making any major changes to your usual lifestyle. The suggestions in this book are based on the latest scientific and medical findings, and such findings make conclusions as to what's best for the average person. But every person is unique. A nutritional or exercise principle that works fine for most people may not always be best for you. Therefore, always check with your physician first.

Now let's see how you'll look and feel better from the very first day you begin to practice what you read. These fifty-two ways really can work to slow your biological clock!

PART I

Shape Your Body With Exercise

We're starting off with exercise, because this and nutrition (in part II) are the easiest areas for people to slip up on as they grow older, and also the quickest in which you can see improvement when you start doing more sensible things. With better exercise and nutrition, you can almost instantly sense your health, vigor, and well-being improve. This is no exaggeration—literally within a day, you should notice pronounced enhancement in mood, self-concept, alertness, and how you feel overall. To make sure you do it right and don't overdo it, we'll start off in chapter 1 with stretching, probably the most overlooked of all techniques to improve your vigor and reverse the signs of aging.

Stretch for Life

Since his teenage years, Charles has always loved to hike and jog. But around thirty-five years of age, he began to notice gradually worsening aches and pains from exercise and routine physical activities such as carrying groceries. Once he tore something in his right heel, developing plantar fascitis, and couldn't run for months. The doctors prescribed rest, hot or cold compresses, and medications to fight the tissue inflammation. He went through a lot of ibuprofen and other pain medications in an attempt to find relief.

Then he read a book on sports injuries and learned that his heel problem was caused by a failure to properly stretch the calf muscles prior to running. After just a few days of careful but brief stretching, his poor heel began to mend and feel better. Later, when he started getting hip pains and backaches, he again discovered that proper stretching could solve the problem.

Don't consider such aches and pains to be typical and inevitable in the aging process. You, too, can lessen or eliminate such problems through the simple act of stretching your muscles, ligaments, and tendons, which otherwise would grow tighter with age. By counteracting this process, you can move and feel like someone years or even decades younger! You can bust this sign of age.

Before You Start

- First, learn to distinguish whether your own hurts and discomforts stem from simple lack of flexibility or true degenerative conditions requiring more complex treatment. For instance, rheumatoid arthritis inflames the joints and makes movement painful but requires professional medical treatment rather than just more stretching. Consult your physician if you have any doubt.

- If you've been losing flexibility for many years now, remember to start stretching at only a very modest level and build up only very gradually. Otherwise, you'll almost certainly injure yourself and wind up worse off than you are now. It took years or even decades for you to lose your flexibility. You won't gain it back in just a few days. So take your time.

- Never stretch to the point of pain. Some people have heard the motto "No pain, no gain" and think that they're supposed to strain themselves until they really hurt or else the workout is useless. Wrong! It's just the opposite—pushing yourself to the point of real pain will likely result in injuries, which will prevent you from gaining the flexibility you need. Instead, stretch just to the point where you feel resistance or a kind of tug, which is no more than slightly uncomfortable at worst. Done right, stretching should feel good while you do it and afterward.

- Stretch slowly and gradually, especially for the first few months of stretching. You've probably seen very flexible people do so-called ballistic stretches in which they bounce rapidly into a highly stretched position. For instance, some people can bounce in a touch-your-toes maneuver all the way down until their flat palms touch the floor. Any beginner trying this is going to tear something, and it will be very painful and prevent all stretching for some time. Don't even try it!

- Stretch regularly. Develop a plan that fits your lifestyle and stick with it. If you can, stretch every day or almost every day. More often (twice a day, for example) probably won't help you any more than once a day. If you're engaging in strenuous exercise hours after your last stretch period ended, however, it might be good to do a little stretching just before and after.

- How long should you stretch? How much time can you afford? One minute is better than none. Ten minutes is better than five. You can do a complete workout as described below in twenty to thirty minutes, but that's not essential every day. Adapt the plan to your schedule and don't worry if the session length varies a bit from day to day. Do five repetitions one day and only two another day if you're running late. But don't do five repetitions of half the stretches and then none of the other half.

- Where should you stretch? Buy an exercise mat or place a soft towel over your carpet. If you stretch on a surface that's too hard, you'll probably get sore, or even bruised.

- One final point—just prior to stretching exercises, spend a minute or two warming up. Before standing up, try the human equivalent of the "doggie stretch" (think of the way canines stretch the whole body from head to tail when they first get up after a rest). In other words, lean back with your arms in the air, tense the muscles, then extend your arms all the way up. Take a big breath and feel your torso stretch. Then send tension rippling down your legs, from hips to toes. Next, stand up and massage your arms and legs briefly, shake out your limbs, and maybe run in place for a few steps. This prepares your body for the exercise to come. And remember to cool down afterward.

Basic Stretching Maneuvers

You don't have to do all of these every day, but you might want to try them all at least once and then decide which ones to keep. Or you could do some one day and then others the next, rotating back and forth. For maximum benefit, however, you should do at least some from each of the three categories in every session.

Arm Stretches

- *Elbow lifts.* Stand with your fists at your chest and your elbows at your sides. Gradually raise your elbows up perpendicular to your body, then release.

- *Shoulder stretch.* Next, hold your hands, fingers interlaced, at the back of your neck with elbows straight in front. Slightly raise your elbows up, then release. Then gradually roll your elbows back until they're parallel with your shoulders, and release.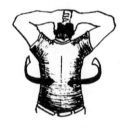

- *Triceps stretch.* Bend one arm so that your elbow points straight up, with that hand loose behind your head. With your other hand, grab the elbow and pull it slightly toward your head until you feel the triceps (back of the upper arm) stretch. Release and repeat with your other arm.

Back Flexibility and Strength

- *Pelvic tilt.* Lie flat on your back on the mat with your knees bent as shown. Flatten the curve of your back against the floor by tightening your stomach and buttocks and pushing the top of your pelvis backward. Hold for about three seconds, then repeat.

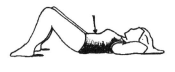

- *One knee to chest.* Lie flat on your back with your knees bent. Grasp one knee with both hands and pull it toward your chest. Hold for three seconds, then release and repeat with your other knee.

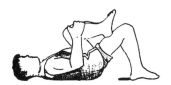

- *Both knees to chest.* In the same position, grasp both knees with your hands and pull them to your chest together. Hold for three seconds, then repeat.

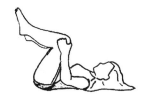

- *Crunches.* On your back, with your knees bent, feet on the floor, and arms across your chest, slowly perform a few partial sit-ups. Make sure you suck in your stomach as those muscles contract.

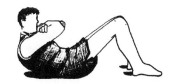

- *Lower trunk rotation.* Flat on your back and with your arms stretched out perpendicular to your body, knees bent, raise

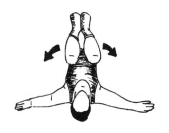

your legs by bending the knees toward your chest. Then rotate your lower trunk slowly side to side.

- *Back bend.* Roll over with your stomach on the floor, legs straight out, arms at your sides. Tuck your chin toward your chest and lift your head, trunk, and arms up off the floor for a few inches. Hold for five seconds, lower to the floor gradually, and then repeat.

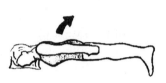

- *Alternate arm and leg lift.* On your stomach, stretch your arms out straight ahead. Gradually lift your right arm and left leg simultaneously for a few inches. Hold for five seconds and gradually lower them. Then repeat with your left arm and right leg.

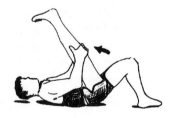

Leg Stretches

- *Hamstring stretch.* Lying on your back with both knees bent, grasp behind one knee and straighten that leg up into the air until you feel a stretch. Hold for fifteen to twenty seconds, and then repeat with your other leg.

- *Thigh stretch.* Lie on your left side. Grab your right heel or the top of your foot and pull it toward your buttocks, bending at the knee. Hold for fifteen to twenty seconds, then roll over to your other side and repeat with your other leg. You can also strengthen your hip muscles by staying on your side and slowly raising your free leg off the floor several inches.

- *Hip stretch.* Lie on back with bent knees but with your legs far apart, feet on the floor. Contract your stomach slightly to force your lower back down against the floor, and roll your knees toward each other slowly without moving your feet. Release slowly, and then repeat.

- *Calf stretch.* Stand with your hands against a wall, with your left leg about eighteen inches farther from the wall than your right. Keep your left heel flat on the floor and that knee straight, then slowly bend forward until your calf stretches. Hold for five seconds, then release and repeat with the other leg.

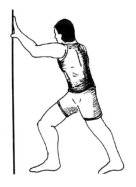

The Benefits of Stretching

Sticking with a regular stretching program for just a few minutes every day or so can preserve youthful flexibility, decrease the risk of injuries, and ensure that you recover more readily if an injury should occur.

Stretch for life!

CHAPTER 2

Take Up Heart-Smart Exercise

Research has proven time and again that even a little exercise on a regular basis can add years to your life. Even people in their sixties and seventies who have been out of shape for decades can improve their health, strength, vigor, mental acuity, and happiness with moderate exercise. But please notice that word *moderate*. Among people who are severely out of shape and suddenly decide to exercise all-out, like they did when younger, almost all will hurt themselves; a few may collapse from heart attacks and even die. So please be sensible: first consult your physician, then start a very modest level and only very gradually work your way up to more intense sessions. Begin any vigorous workout by stretching with the exercises we talked about in chapter 1. Always cool down and stretch afterward as well.

Pick the Exercises Best for You

Selecting something you enjoy, whether team sports or solo activities, makes it easier to stick with exercise on a regular basis. If you truly hate jogging, for example, what's the point in starting? Better to choose physical activities you really like and will stick with, whether it's tennis or riding a bike.

The only rule is to pick something that gets your body moving to the point where your heart and breathing rates are noticeably picking up and staying up. The same endeavor may or may not count as real exercise, depending upon how vigorously you do it. Gardening, for instance, can be too light to really count, or it can be energetic. If you sit still for minutes at a time while lightly weeding, it won't give you much of a workout. But the day you spend walking to and fro, carrying and spreading fertilizer and seeds and so forth, is a different story. So you could garden vigorously some days, and on your easy gardening days you could play handball or swim.

Always Protect Your Heart

If your exercise gets too intense and your heart starts to skip beats, race, or otherwise seems to be straining, quit! Listen to your body and be safe. In order to check your heart rate, take your pulse during exercise, either at the wrist or the carotid artery in the side of your neck. A full minute provides the most accurate count. But it's more convenient to count for fifteen seconds and then multiply by four, or even count for six seconds and multiply by ten for a beats-per-minute estimate. Here are some guidelines for a safe target range of your heartbeat during exercise as a function of your age. But these are averages only. If these heart rates strain you, slow down.

Your maximum heart rate is generally about 220 beats per minute, minus your age. If you're 50, for example, that works out to $220 - 50 = 170$. If you're 30, that works out to 190. But this isn't your target—it's the point at which you're risking death! Your target during exercise should only be 60 to 70 percent of your theoretical maximum. So for a person who's 50, that works out to 60 percent of $170 = 102$, while 70 percent of $170 = 119$. So the target range is about 102 to 119 beats per minute. As you get more fit over time, you can safely go a bit higher than 70 percent, but we don't recommend this early on. Rather than calculate this exactly for yourself, you can consult the simplified table below, which is provided by the National Heart, Lung, and Blood Institute. This table allows an upward boundary of 75 percent of your maximum heart rate, for when you get more fit.

Exercise Heart Rate to Aim For

AGE	DESIRABLE HEART-RATE RANGE
20	120–150
25	117–146
30	114–142
35	111–138
40	108–135
45	105–131
50	102–127
55	99–123
60	96–120
65	Consult your physician for a heart checkup before choosing and calculating a safe percent of your maximum, or before starting an exercise program

Twelve Ways to Get more Active

To achieve any long-term benefit from exercise, it's important to work out at least two or three days a week. Up to once or twice a day is fine, too, unless your body begins to complain about it. But don't think of exercise only as formal, scheduled periods for specific activities. Rather, strive gradually to become more active in all areas of your life, even when sitting at a desk at work. Here are some possibilities:

1. Get off the subway or bus one stop before yours and walk the extra half mile or mile.

2. Park farther from your building and walk more.

3. Take the stairs, not the elevator. (If you're in a tall building and twenty-six floors are too many to walk, take the elevator up to, say, two or three floors below yours, then walk the rest of the way.)

4. Use your coffee break for a ten-minute walk through or around your building.

5. When you see someone else lifting or moving items, volunteer to help.

6. Do isometric exercises at your desk. These are exercises in which you push or pull against nonmoving objects. For instance, while sitting, grab the arms of your chair and rhythmically tug and pull in a variety of different directions, one at a time. Make sure you balance this each session by feeling the tug in all the muscles of your arms.

7. Cut your lawn with a walking power mower rather than a rider.

8. Use hand clippers to trim the bushes rather than power clippers. The same goes for sawing, digging, and all sorts of yard work or other handiwork.

9. Think of household chores such as sweeping and mopping as opportunities for exercise rather than bores.

10. When you plan to visit friends or relatives who live close by, consider a hike rather than a drive to see them.

11. When you let the dog out, don't just stand there with a coffee cup watching. Put him on a leash and escort him on a royal tour of all the bushes and trees.

12. If you have only minor shopping at the corner store, walk there and back rather than cranking up the car.

Build Muscle

A well-rounded exercise program includes not only stretching and aerobic activities to develop your heart and lungs, but also muscle-building workouts. Without them, our muscles tend slowly and gradually to diminish in size and grow weaker as we get older. For instance, muscle mass seriously starts to drop off after age fifty-five, with strength declining about 15 percent in our sixties, another 15 percent in our seventies, and then 30 percent per decade after that. Then if we suddenly try to do something we could easily do when younger—say, heft the lawn mower into the car to take it in for repairs—we can't readily do it. If we try to force ourselves, we may instead cause an injury.

A really good muscle-building program requires weight sets or other gym equipment. People who feel strongly committed to pursue this would be well advised to either join a gym that has equipment available or buy their own for home use. (But please don't get gung-ho in the beginning, spend a fortune on home equipment, give up using it after two weeks, then get mad at yourself for wasting money and clogging up living space.)

There are good alternatives to spending a lot on equipment:

- Do strengthening exercises that don't require special gear, such as calisthenics (push-ups, sit-ups, squats).

- Borrow a friend's sports paraphernalia to make sure you enjoy it before buying your own.

- Use common household items as weights to see if you'll be able to stick to a regular program before you buy gym weights. For example, try doing arm curls and rotations while holding a can of food in each hand. Try doing squats while holding a jug of water in each hand. Two cautions here, however. First, household items aren't compact weights and don't have the right kind of handles for exercise, so you're more prone to injury with any but fairly light (for you) weights. Second, it will be difficult to gradually increase weight as you get stronger.

More muscle makes you look younger and more vigorous. It keeps the metabolic rate up and helps you burn more calories twenty-four hours a day. In fact, your body must burn an extra thirty to fifty calories a day for each pound of lean muscle. Zapping those extra calories keeps you trimmer and slimmer, more content with your body and appearance. If you do develop a serious weight-lifting program, however, be sure to eat sufficient protein (see chapters 5 and 11) and also vitamin E. A study at the Human Performance Laboratory at Ball State University, just reported in 2001, found that men engaging in fifty-minute weight-lifting work-outs experienced less muscle damage if they ingested more than the typical recommended daily intake of vitamin E. The re-searchers recommended up to 1,200 international units (IU) daily—but only for serious weight lifters, and only those not also taking blood thinners. People using weights only occasionally for minor muscle toning (say, five to ten minutes a time, two or three times a week) have not demonstrated a need for more than usual (see chapter 15) vitamin E.

Don't let your muscles progressively deteriorate with age. Studies have shown that people in their sixties, seventies, and even eighties who haven't exercised regularly for decades can success-fully rebuild at least some of their muscle. The Honolulu Heart Program, which has been studying the health of eight thousand men since 1965, reported in the *New England Journal of Medicine* that those older men who walked a couple of miles a day cut their risk of death almost in half compared to the less active elderly men. It doesn't seem fair, but when you're out of shape you burn fewer calories, which makes you tend to stay out of shape. But the oppo-site is true, too. Once you get in shape, it's easier to stay thin, be-cause all those extra muscles just keep burning away your calories!

To keep up with the latest information for strengthening and protecting your heart, consult the American Heart Association's Web site: www.americanheart.org.

CHAPTER 3

Hike for Health

M any folks dread the thought of working out at a gym in front of other people or putting on an athletic costume and running down the street. But unless you suffer from leg injuries, the one exercise you can always rely on is walking. You don't have to dress fancy or spend money on equipment. You can do it alone or with company. You can listen to music on a Sony Walkman, talk to a friend, take the dog, admire the beauties of nature, or just wander off lost in thought. (If you take music, do keep it low enough that you can still remain aware of your surroundings.)

However you do it, get out there and take a trek. Ease on down the road. Hike the highway. Pump the pavement. Stride down the street. Even tiptoe through the tulips. Whatever you want to call it, just get out and do it!

The Amazing Benefits of Walking

Just sidling from your easy chair to the car doesn't cut it. But if you get outside and walk vigorously for at least fifteen or twenty minutes, to the point where your heart and breathing rates noticeably pick up, you can expect advantages like these:

- *You'll strengthen your heart, lungs, and bones.* Walking only once a month won't improve anything, but regular walking at least two or three times a week will help keep your old ticker ticking. Your heart will pump blood more efficiently, your lungs will process air more effectively, and your bones will grow stronger, more resistant to exercise stress. You'll get in better shape generally, with your leg muscles in particular noticeably toning up.

- *You'll feel better.* As you get back into physical shape, you'll feel more energetic, more awake, more alive. Any kind of vigorous exercise, including walking, makes the brain release marvelous chemicals called endorphins, which heighten your sense of well-being and pleasure in life.

- *You'll ease tension.* After a hard day at work, commuting through road rage, or wrestling with problems at home, walking makes a good stress release. The tension just seems to melt away with every minute of physical activity.

- *You'll think more clearly.* When you feel better physically and emotionally, when stress loses its grip on you, you'll begin to think more clearly. You're more likely to arrive at answers for your questions and solutions for your problems. Scientific studies prove that people at work perform better and more creatively if they use breaks for brief walks.

- *You'll burn calories.* Every mile burns about a hundred calories. So walking five miles per week, for example, uses about five hundred calories. At that rate, you could burn off a pound of fat in about seven weeks. If you build up to five miles per day, you could burn that next pound of fat in just seven days. Plus, as we discussed last chapter, every bit of muscle you build through exercise will keep burning calories throughout the entire day, even when you're not exercising.

- *You'll suppress your appetite.* Not only does a good walk burn more calories, but it also helps control your appetite so that you tend to eat less—and tend to eat a healthier diet. Want to control those cravings for chocolate or potato chips? Try a good walk or other exercise instead. You'll lose weight. And keep it off.

- *You'll reduce health risks.* Being obese and sedentary leads you toward all sorts of disease hazards such as heart disease, cancer, and diabetes. Such afflictions can slash years off your life. But regular walking or other exercise helps keep your weight down and strengthen your system against such diseases. You won't live forever, but you'll probably live longer. And you'll enjoy those extra years a whole lot more. One of the best controlled exercise studies ever done was conducted by the University of Helsinki in Finland. Researchers studied sixteen thousand twins for an average of nineteen years, in order to separate out the effects of heredity on longevity from those of exercise. The twins who took walks at least six times a month for half an hour each time cut their risk of death by 44 percent compared to their brothers or sisters who remained inactive. Clearly, walking has very beneficial effects on health whether your genes are good or bad.

Do It Right

- Remember to stretch before and after, as discussed in chapter 1.

- Wear good shoes that both feel comfortable and provide traction.

- Drink some fluids before and after your walk, or even during the walk if it's a long one.

- Don't walk too far or keep walking if part of your leg or foot hurts—you don't want to create or worsen an injury.

- Unless you're in primo shape, don't walk with hand or ankle weights. Ankle weights can throw off your gait and risk injury.

Hey . . . Be Careful Out There!

- Be mindful of the weather and dress appropriately. You don't want to get a chill from underdressing or grow overheated from overdressing. It's okay to walk even in bad weather such as rain or snow, provided you dress suitably. Use multiple layers when it's cold; you can remove one or more as you heat up during exercise.

- Choose as safe a trail as you can, avoiding high-traffic areas or other hazards such as potholes or excess debris. If you live in an area where crime is a concern, avoid areas too secluded or unused. A walking or running trail is ideal if you live near one. If you don't, try the perimeter around a nearby park, lake, or something similar. If all else fails, walk on the city sidewalks, but be careful when crossing streets.

- In the dark, don't walk outside without a flashlight. And use reflective clothing if your trail crosses vehicular traffic at any point.

- Watch out for slick and slippery spots formed by ice, mud, grease, oil, or green, moist lichen. Once Charles was walking on a sidewalk in the predawn hours and slipped on an invisible ice patch. His feet flew into the air and he fell on the pavement flat on his back before he knew what was happening! Thankfully, he sustained only some minor cuts and bruises rather than broken bones.

Avoid Indoor Hazards, Too

- A good treadmill is your best bet, but it can be rather costly. If you use one, follow the manufacturer's instructions regarding placement and use. Beware of going too fast or mounting or dismounting carelessly so that you slip off the tread while it's still moving.

- Without equipment it's possible to walk for twenty minutes indoors even in a small home or apartment, but it can get rather boring. Clear the clutter in the rooms you'll use. Then watch for furniture as you pace back and forth, to and fro, up and down stairs. Better yet, take an indoor walk in a large public building or mall. Some malls have indoor walking trails marked out.

Walking is fun and it feels good. Make that a regular part of your lifestyle. You won't regret it!

CHAPTER 4

Breathe Healthy and Relax

You might assume breathing is so automatic that you don't need to think about it. Not so. Before birth, all of our bodily organs are formed, including the lungs. But while the others work normally even within the mother's womb (the heart beats, the ears hear), the lungs, of course, don't take in air. Sometimes babies have difficulty taking that first breath of real air after birth—hence the quick spank on the bottom to get them started.

Basic breathing among us is automatic and requires no conscious thought, of course, hence we can breathe while asleep and even unconscious. Still, various conditions can alter our breathing pattern and make it less efficient. Sometimes conscious and deliberate breathing is called for, not to maintain life, but to enhance mental alertness and emotional well-being.

Things That Can Mess Up Breathing

Various emotional states can really throw off your breathing. Have you ever been very tense and noticed a tautness in your chest? It felt as if someone had a stretch band around your chest and was squeezing it tighter and tighter. Have you ever been nervous or anxious and noticed that your breathing was shallow and rapid, and that you were getting a little light-headed? Sometimes people get fearful or even panic and lose all control over their breathing. They hyperventilate with rapid, shallow, almost gasping breaths.

Breathing like this will ensure enough oxygen to maintain life, but it doesn't feel very good. It actually adds to your distress in a vicious circle. The more nervous you are, the worse you breathe. The worse you breathe, the more nervous and upset you become. And so on.

Break the Nervous Cycle

You can jump out of this vicious spiral by regaining control over your breathing. A good time to practice this is when you're falling asleep, trying to return to sleep after being awakened, or taking a brief rest break at work (as covered in chapter 36). It's really very simple, but it takes some practice.

- Get into as comfortable a position as you can, hopefully away from distractions and with your eyes closed.

- Become aware of your breathing. Concentrate on it, think about it, analyze it. Is your breathing rapid, high up in your lungs, or shallow?

- Deliberately change your breathing pattern. Assert control.

- Begin to breathe from deep in your abdomen rather than high up in your chest. When you're tense, you'll probably notice primarily your chest heaving in and out. That way, it's mostly your upper lungs that get the air. Instead, force your diaphragm—low in your abdomen—to move down and out. You should sense that your lower stomach area is doing more work than your chest. Now you should be filling all your lungs well with air.

- Start breathing regularly. No more gasping or panting. No more jagged breaths or other irregularities. The easiest way is to count slowly while breathing in, say a count of five or ten, then make the same count while breathing out. Pause a moment before exhaling and also again between breaths.

- Breathe more slowly. If you breathe deeply and at a deliberate, regular rate, you should be able to slow down your breathing. You become more efficient as you exert less effort to more fully oxygenate your lungs.

- If you start hyperventilating, breathe into a small paper bag. This way you breathe back in some of your own carbon dioxide, the chemical balance of which signals your brain to start breathing normally again.

When you breathe deeply, regularly, and slowly, you should notice an almost immediate release of tension and a sharp increase in mental alertness. It's as if you were suddenly getting pulses of enriched oxygen directly into the brain. Next time you're about to enter a stressful situation, perhaps public speaking or confronting an angry customer, try this out and see if it doesn't help you conquer your anxiety.

Proper breathing can even help control pain. Controlling breathing is a major component of handling the stress of natural childbirth, for instance.

Breathing is essential for life. And better breathing makes life better. Breathe healthy and relax!

PART II

Build Your Body With Diet and Nutrition

Now that we've talked about how to burn calories, let's discuss more fully the intake side of the calorie equation. We'll devote several chapters to what types of food you should minimize, then focus on the ones you should emphasize in a healthy diet. The latter chapters include mouthwatering recipes to make sure you have foods you can really enjoy as well as enhance health with.

CHAPTER 5

Cut a Few Pounds

Does your weight worry you? Surveys reveal that most people say yes. Either we really are too fat or we think we are when we aren't. The most extreme example of this is the anorexic girl who starves herself into a dangerously thin state—yet still looks into a mirror and thinks she's fat. So first you should figure out if you really do need to lose a few pounds. Try to be objective about this.

How to Know if You Should Lose Weight

There are several ways to approach this problem. Let's start with a few informal ones.

Rough Estimate Techniques

- Can you "pinch an inch"? Sit upright in a chair, relax your abdomen, and pinch your belly. Do you get more than an inch in that pinch? If so, maybe you should consider losing some of what you just tweaked.

- In adulthood, have you had to buy larger clothing sizes over the years or had to expand your belt to looser notches? If so, maybe your clothes are trying to tell you something.

- Get a tape measure and assess your waist and hip sizes. If your waist is the larger of the two for both men and women, it's time to reduce—unless, of course, you're pregnant.

- Do you jiggle noticeably when walking rapidly or running? If the answer is yes, that's another warning for you.

Official Techniques

- Check a height/weight chart for your sex to see if you exceed the recommended guidelines (see the table on the opposite page).

- See your doctor if you have any doubt about whether you could stand to lose some weight. Medical professionals are able to take precise measurements with instruments or calculate your body mass index (BMI) or even do other tests to discern if those pounds on your bathroom scale are bone and muscle or actually excess fat.

The Advantages of Weight Loss

Let's assume one or more of the above tests yields bad news (after all, most of us really are overweight these days). Is it best just to ignore the problem? Simply "eat, drink, and be merry"? Few remember the rest of this saying: "for tomorrow we die."

Being overweight does threaten to damage your health and cut your life span short. And the more overweight you are, the worse are the results. It may be fun to put on those excess pounds by chomping on cheesecake and chocolate chip cookies. But the excess flab slows you down, makes accidents more likely to happen, increases the risk of heart disease, strokes, diabetes, and other killer illnesses, hurts your appearance, and impairs your social and emotional health.

Aren't these reasons enough?

Healthy Weight Ranges for Adult Men and Women of All Ages

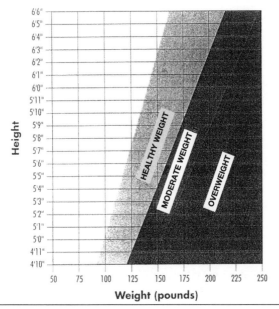

SOURCE: *Living Smart* brochure, © 1999, American Cancer Society, Inc. Created by the National Institute of Medicine.

Lose Weight Safely

Okay. You realize you're overweight and you want to do something about it for your health's sake. Now what? Pay close attention, because many people go about losing weight the wrong way, some even risking their health more than if they'd kept the extra pounds.

- *Shun fad diets.* Forget about all those impossible-to-be-true diet claims. Don't even experiment with an unbalanced diet that leaves out one or more of the basic food groups (protein, dairy, fruits, vegetables, and grains). Sure, you can lose weight by eating nothing or an extreme diet centered on only

one kind of food—but you could also lose your health. Many
have fallen sick and a few have even died by forsaking dietary
balance.

- *Lose weight gradually.* If you try to lose too much, too fast, it
  only means that you're depriving yourself. You'll probably
  feel bad, quit soon, regain all the lost weight, and usually add
  another pound or two when the diet ends. Additionally, rapid
  weight loss usually means that muscle and body water have
  dropped off rather than fat.

- *Slowly change your caloric intake-output balance.* Just re-
  stricting caloric intake is like driving to work with one hand
  tied behind your back—difficult at best, and downright risky
  to boot. But if you reduce your intake only slightly while also
  boosting output through exercise, you'll be more likely to
  consume enough nutrients for health, good mood, and vigor
  while protecting your muscle mass, reshaping your body, and
  ensuring fat loss. Pretty cool, eh?

- *Make changes you can live with.* Most people planning a diet
  decide to give up all their desserts, snacks, favorite foods,
  and comfort yum-yums. After a day or two, they feel so deprived that they jump off the wagon. Then they gorge on
  treats and feel guilty and resolve to quit better next time . . .
  and so on, in a constant cycle. Avoid this yo-yo lifestyle!
  Make dietary and exercise changes that you can live with
  permanently. Better to make a small lasting change than a
  large one that you quickly give up.

- *Suppress appetite with color.* Have you ever noticed that
  fast-food restaurants tend to be decorated with bright colors
  such as orange, yellow, or red? Bright colors tend to enhance
  the appetite. Reverse this principle to help suppress your
  appetite: when you eat, do so in a room or area with darker
  colors.

How to Lose Weight and Keep It Off

Mild Dietary Restriction

Think of this not as a "diet" but rather as a "new eating plan." You really can eat anything you like and want, but you do need to avoid excess intake. Before eating treats and junk food, therefore, ensure healthy portion sizes of balanced nutritional foods. Most experts recommend daily:

- Two to four servings of fruit (one serving equals one whole apple, banana, or the like; half a cup of mixed fruit pieces; or three-quarters of a cup of juice).

- Three to five servings of vegetables (each half a cup if cooked or chopped, but one cup for leafy raw veggies like lettuce). Make sure at least one of these servings is of high-protein veggies such as beans or peas.

- Six to ten servings of grain (one serving is one slice of bread, one roll, one ounce of dry cereal, or half a cup of cooked cereal, pasta, or rice).

- Two to three servings of dairy products such as milk (one cup each), cheese (two ounces each), or yogurt.

- One to two servings of protein foods such as meat, poultry, or fish (where one portion is just three or four ounces). Forget about sixteen-ounce steaks!

If you're still hungry after all that, have a snack or two. But keep them small, and be sure to fill up with lots of water.

Mild Increase in Exercise

Check with your physician *before* starting any exercise plan if you've been out of shape and have not exercised for several months or years. Then start at a very mild level and work your way up very, very gradually, as discussed in chapter 2.

Every time you work out those muscles—however you do it—you're burning calories. Researchers at NASA studied five hundred NASA employees over ten years and found that those who exercised regularly didn't gain weight over that decade even if they didn't improve their eating habits. How much better if you do both!

Weight loss really is as simple as eating fewer calories and burning more of them. In future chapters, we'll share more ideas on improving your diet, reducing items that aren't so healthy (chapters 6 through 9) and increasing intake of the good stuff (chapters 10 through 19).

CHAPTER 6

Learn to Be Jack Spratt

Jack Spratt could eat no fat,
His wife could eat no lean,
And so betwixt them both, you see,
They licked the platter clean.

—Mother Goose rhyme

Though some fad diets disagree, we believe that the number one secret to a healthful, low-calorie eating plan is to reduce dietary fat. Why? Because fat contains more calories than any other nutrient in the food chain. Thus, a serving of a high-fat food may not satisfy hunger any better than one of a low-fat food, but it will burden your system with far more calories. Also, high fat intake leads to negative health consequences like an increase in the bad cholesterol that can clog your arteries and cause all sorts of life-threatening diseases.

Moreover, dietary fat is converted into your own body fat a lot more readily than the same number of calories from any other nutrient. Your body has to really work to chemically transform excess protein or carbohydrate into body fat. But it requires far less energy merely to move incoming fat from your digestive tract out to the layers of blubber stored in your body.

Recognize Fat in Foods

Watch out for two problems in reducing dietary fat. First of all, fat generally tastes good. Most people prefer tossed salad, for instance, with a fatty salad dressing slathered on top. We like baked potatoes smothered in butter or cheese—both sources of fat.

But the even greater obstacle may be a lack of awareness of how fat hides in so many foods. Trimming highly visible layers of fat off a steak or pork chop still leaves hundreds of fat calories in the remaining meat. Not all fat is visible—much hides at the microscopic level in cell membranes and within the cells of the meat. There's simply no way at home to remove it all.

Other fat conceals itself in the form of oils, which are just about 100 percent fat. Take peanuts and other nuts, for example. Nuts have lots of protein and carbohydrates and useful vitamins and minerals. They would be an ideal food—except that they're full of fatty oil, which provides about three-quarters of their calories! Even certain fruits like avocados are fairly high in fat. One hint: if a food is known also for its oil (such as olive oil or peanut oil), then that food contains loads of fat.

Processed foods actually add even more fat. As if there weren't already enough fat in chocolate, when they make cake they add more fat (butter, shortening) during preparation. Ditto for potato chips and all manner of processed desserts, snacks, and treats. We know, we know—these foods taste great. We like them, too. No one is saying you must shun them entirely, but do take it easy!

Reduce Fat in Your Eating Plan

Eliminate High-Fat Foods You Can Do Without

Don't eat any high-fat food you can live without. Years ago, we gave up mayonnaise when making sandwiches. They tasted a little different at first, but it was no big hardship for us to make this change. Avoiding fatty foods you don't really want allows you to enjoy the ones you truly crave. Yet with moderation, you can still remain on the healthy eating plan.

Reduce Portion Size or Frequency of Cherished Fatty Foods

It's going to be tougher to restrict intake of the fatty foods you really care about. Don't try to eliminate them entirely, but do cut down. Either eat them as frequently as usual but cut down on portion size, *or* keep the usual portion size but consume them less frequently.

For example, if now you eat about four ounces of potato chips each evening after dinner, that's too much. Either cut down to, say, one ounce a day, or continue to eat four but do so only once a week, perhaps as a treat on Friday night. If you still feel hungry during your usual snack time, then eat something low in fat, like pretzels, carrot or celery sticks, or some fruit.

Cutting down may not be fun, but it can be done. Carlota loves avocados and could readily eat them at every meal. Instead she has them only about once a month. Charles loves eggs and grew up eating two every morning. Now he only has three or four a week. Such foods aren't entirely bad for you, of course; they also contain some great nutrients, such as vitamins in the avocados and protein and choline in the eggs. Such high-fat foods may be good for you in moderation, but try to keep it that way.

Choose Tasty Low-Fat Substitutions

Sometimes you really can't give up a cherished food that's fatty without a nagging sense of deprivation. In such cases, substitute something else lower in fat that tastes almost as good. For instance, how many people could stand to eat a plain baked potato? But each tablespoon of butter you spread in adds about a hundred calories and nine grams of fat. Instead, try light sour cream, which adds only twenty calories and one and a quarter grams of fat—far less. Better yet, dispense with fat altogether by adding just a few sprinkles of garlic powder and parsley! Experiment to find the spice blend that appeals most to you.

Similarly, if you don't like to eat tossed green salad plain, instead of drowning your lettuce in a high-fat dressing, try light dollops of one low in fat or even fat-free. Select milk with the greatest reduction in fat you can stand, preferably 1 percent fat milk, ½ percent fat, or even skim.

What about special reduced-fat snack products? Don't rely on these as the solution. Studies show that people who depend on these often develop a worse diet than before. Why? They see the *reduced-fat* label, consider the food nutritionally safe, and then eat *more* sweets and junk than before!

Prepare Low-Fat Meals

- Buy leaner cuts of meat.

- Always trim off and discard visible fat from ham, beef, pork, and other meats.

- Whenever possible, bake or grill foods rather than frying them.

- When you must fry, use as little oil as possible, and choose one low in saturated fat (such as olive oil).

- Discard the fat released during cooking. For example, when frying bacon, toss out all the liquid lard produced. When roasting, allow the juices to cool in the refrigerator and skim off the solid white fat that forms on the top. The remaining gelatin contains more protein than fat and makes a nice gravy when reheated.

Learn to eat like Jack Spratt, and you'll look and feel a whole lot healthier!

CHAPTER 7

Sidestep Your Sweet Tooth

"How sweet it is!"
"Kisses sweeter than wine."
"Sweet victory."

Our culture considers the word *sweet* as a veritable synonym for *good*. During the hunter-gatherer phase of humankind, there was a certain logic to that. Even now, if a wild plant tastes sweet, it's probably safe to eat. If it tastes bitter, it probably contains druglike compounds, which can often be toxic.

But in a culture where the supermarket offers thousands of food products to choose from, a sweet taste is often used to bolster one's competitive edge. Thus, sugar is added to hundreds of food products, many of which don't fit into the "dessert" or "treat" category at all. As if that weren't enough, we buy sugar in big five-pound bags and ladle it into coffee, tea, and other beverages. We sprinkle it over cereal and pour it by the pound into batters for cookies and cakes. We gorge on candy, pies, ice cream, and other sweets such as pancakes or waffles swimming in syrup. As a result, modern Americans are practically drowning in sugar. The average American consumes about 135 pounds of sugar per year! That's way too much.

Negative Effects of Excess Sugar Intake

- *Tooth decay.* One of the most obvious effects of sugar overload is on the teeth, about which we'll have more to say in chapter 22. Let it suffice here to point out that before the discovery of sugar refining, people had less tooth decay than now. That's right! Primitive humans lived out their days with better teeth than many of us modern people have, even with all our fluoridated water, toothpaste, toothbrushes, and dentists. And purified sugar appearing in countless foods is the main reason for this difference. The bacteria always found in the mouth just love sugar—they thrive on it and produce the acids that eat away at the protective enamel on our teeth.

- *Weight gain.* Sugar adds a lot to the average person's caloric load and is another reason for the outbreak of obesity in our time. Every gram of pure sugar adds four calories. So a pound of sugar brings in about eighteen hundred calories! If you're watching your weight, eighteen hundred calories is in the ballpark of one day's total recommended intake. Yet a lot of people consume close to that much in sugar alone.

- *Displacement of healthier fare.* Have you ever seen kids rush home from school ravenous for a snack? But after a candy bar or two, they aren't hungry when it's time for dinner. Pure sugar does provide energy, but that's all it does. It doesn't give you any other kind of nutrition, neither vitamins nor minerals. And to the extent that you fill up on it, you're avoiding foods such as complex carbohydrates that do provide the nutrition your body craves. Sugarholics simply won't get the recommended daily amounts of protein foods, fruits, and vegetables after they've gorged on sugar products.

- *Increased risk of disease.* Excessive sugar is linked to a number of diseases, most notably diabetes, which is one of our biggest killers. There are many factors behind diabetes besides excessive sugar intake, but it certainly does make diabetes worse. In this disease, either the pancreas doesn't produce enough insulin or the body doesn't respond properly to what is produced. Without a good insulin response, the body can't properly control blood sugar levels. Chronic high levels of blood sugar can, over time, cause nerve damage, sexual dysfunction, blindness, and eventually death. If you have diabetes, a history of diabetes in your family, or any other reason to suspect you may be at risk, please avoid uncontrolled sugar intake.

- *Mood effects.* Even in healthy people, excessive sugar intake can screw up the insulin response. As your intestines shoot the extra sugar into your blood, the rising level screams to the pancreas for help. The pancreas obliges by sending out extra insulin in self-defense. If your system doesn't realize how much sugar you've taken in, the body may respond with too much insulin, quickly driving blood sugar to levels below normal. This up-and-down yo-yo effect accounts for the well-known sugar "buzz," followed by weakness, lethargy, fatigue, or even a painful headache. Your mood is more likely to remain steadily up with moderate (or no) purified sugar intake.

Cut Down Your Sugar Intake

Choose Nature's Sweets

We mention purified sugar here to contrast with the various natural sugars already found in most plant foods, particularly fruits. That's why apples, peaches, tangerines, and the like inherently taste sweet. Natural forms of sugar are found in other foods, too, most notably milk. (The lactose in milk, however, doesn't taste very sweet.) To satisfy your craving for sweets, we recommend turning to fruit before you indulge in cake, cookies, pie, ice cream, pudding, candy, and other desserts and sweet treats. We're talking about ordinary fresh fruit here, not fruit slices drowning in heavy sugar syrup or coated with powdered sugar.

Limit Dessert-Type Foods

Sweetened desserts like those just mentioned contain piles of added sugar that your body can readily do without. When you make desserts from scratch at home, you'll recognize instantly from the recipe how much sugar you're adding. With store-bought processed foods, it's not quite so easy. Instead, read the list of ingredients on the label. How many forms of sugar do you see? Look for items such as *sugar, honey, corn syrup, other syrup, glucose, fructose, sucrose,* and other words ending in *-ose.* Remember that all the ingredients are listed in order of how much they contribute to the final product. In other words, the main ingredient in the item is listed first. If, for example, two of the first three items listed are various forms of sugar, then the product in your hand is composed mainly of sugar.

Yes, such foods taste good, and few people could voluntarily give all of them up forever. That's not necessary. But do cut down to moderate amounts that you consume infrequently. Let's say, no more than an ounce or two of sugar once or twice a day, and only after you've eaten some healthy fare first. That's one candy bar, one small slice of cake or pie, or one small bowl of ice cream.

And watch out for sweetened drinks! One can of regular cola contains up to nine teaspoons of sugar—about 150 calories' worth! If you drink one, count it as your dessert, not simply a thirst quencher.

Minimize Artificial Sweeteners

Many people have turned to sodas and other drinks or foods made with artificial sweeteners. On the surface, this seems like the perfect solution. After all, a can of soda with artificial sweeteners contains only a calorie or two at most. What could be better? The reality isn't that simple, however. First, there's considerable controversy over just how safe some artificial sweeteners are, particularly when consumed in large quantities. Second, studies by Robin Kanarek at Tufts University have demonstrated that the use of artificial sweeteners tends to stimulate the appetite and boost overall caloric intake. In reality, people don't simply replace a can of regular soda with diet soda and then shave 150 calories off their total daily intake. Compared to drinking plain water, the diet soda makes them hungrier, and they're more likely to grab that doughnut or second helping of pie. If you feel you must consume such diet foods and drinks, keep this principle in mind and apply even more than usual vigilance over the rest of your daily consumption. Better yet, limit the ingestion of both refined sugar and artificial sweeteners. Not every food or beverage has to taste sweet!

CHAPTER 8

Hide the Saltshaker

Salt doesn't just enhance the flavor of food and help preserve it from spoilage. It's also essential for life. Without salt, your nerves couldn't conduct control signals, and you'd die. In modern society, however, a salt shortage is unthinkable. We are surrounded by salt, in almost every processed food we eat. Many of us also sprinkle it heavily on our food at the table. The average American consumes each day about twenty to thirty times more salt than he or she needs.

Excess salt can be quite dangerous. It gets into your blood along with digested food and draws extra water with it. This tends to increase blood volume and blood pressure, at least among those who are sensitive to this process. Some experts believe that a portion of the public is safe because their kidneys readily excrete all the excess salt. But those unfortunates with a genetic predisposition toward not handling extra salt so completely and promptly can experience serious hypertension (high blood pressure) from today's typically high levels of salt intake. And unless you're sure you're in the safe group, it's a good idea to restrict salt intake any way you comfortably can.

Are You at Risk?

Estimate Your Risk

You're likely in the salt risk group if any or all of the following are true:

- You've ever been measured to have borderline or high blood pressure (above about 140/90).

- Any of your close blood relatives (grandparents, parents, siblings) has ever had hypertension.

- Medical lab tests indicate that your blood sodium (salt) levels tend toward the high end of the scale.

Having any of the above doesn't necessarily mean that you have hypertension now. But it does suggest you may increase your risk for developing this silent killer if you keep ingesting too much salt as you grow older.

The Dangers of Hypertension

Unlike many other diseases, you can have high blood pressure without realizing it. Hypertension can reach even lethal levels without you subjectively having a clue until it's too late. That's one reason why regular checkups are so important. A simple and painless check with the blood pressure cuff will let you and your doctor know what your reading is. If it does come out too high, your physician will suggest further tests, some lifestyle changes (similar to those listed below), and possibly medication to lower the pressure. Without treatment, hypertension can cause dangerous or even lethal heart attacks and strokes, as well as damage to the kidneys and other internal organs.

Ways to Reduce Salt in Your Diet

- *Get rid of the saltshaker.* Go cold turkey if you can. Cut down slowly if you must. But cut down to the point where you never or almost never add salt at the table to your food.

- *Add only the minimum salt during cooking and baking.* If a recipe calls for salt simply to enhance flavor, add the least your taste buds will accept, or replace it altogether with a salt substitute (see below).

- *Minimize processed foods and salty snacks.* Some processed foods include an amazing amount of salt. Look at the ingredient list; odds are that you'll see salt listed, perhaps in several places. For example, it may be listed as prime ingredient and also as an ingredient in each of the subcomponents of the food. Note the *Nutrition Facts* section on the food label. Sodium should be listed, both in terms of amount per serving and also as "%DV" or percent of the suggested Daily Value. If it's more than about 10 to 15 percent of your entire suggested daily intake, consider if you really want your salt in that form, or if a lower-salt food might be just as enjoyable.

    And note especially the serving size. What you actually take as your typical helping may be two to four (or even more) times what the labeled serving size is. In such cases, you would have to multiply the number of servings you plan to eat times the percent of DV. For instance, if six crackers give you 12 percent of your DV, but you actually eat eighteen crackers, that one snack would give you 36 percent of your DV. That's too much!

- *Select fresh, whole foods when possible.* Choose fresh fruit and vegetables for your snacks whenever possible. That's good advice anytime, as pointed out in chapters 10 through 12. Here's another reason—consuming these foods helps keep your salt intake low.

Zesty Alternatives to Salt

Some may complain that they can't give up salt because of the impact on flavor. They won't enjoy their foods, they fear.

Don't worry—there are plenty of alternatives:

- *Salt substitutes.* Table salt is sodium chloride, and the sodium is the troublesome part. Try a salt replacement such as potassium chloride, which provides much of the taste enhancement without any of the sodium.

- *Herbs and spices.* Better yet, try the incredible array of herbs and spices available to jazz up your food without hurting your heart. Consider hot peppers, for instance. As we'll cover in chapter 14, hot peppers (jalapeño, chile, cayenne, and more) not only add zest to food but provide positive health benefits as well. Ditto for garlic, onions, and many others.

In short, reducing salt intake to improve health doesn't mean you must resort to bland, boring food. You can still spice up your life while minimizing salt intake. You owe it to your arteries to do so!

CHAPTER 9

Minimize Artificial Foods

W e've all seen the ads. They come in slightly different forms, but what they boil down to is this: They promise you can lose tons of weight if only you'll give up most or all of your real food and instead consume their "specially formulated" pills, powders, canned drinks, or bars. They promise that their products keep out most of the fat and the calories, but still give you all the nutrients you need to stay healthy and strong. They say you'll even find these powders and potions make "delicious" beverages, and so on.

If all that sounds too good to be true, it basically is. If you cut through all the hype, you'll find a number of problems with these products.

The Limitations of Artificial Foods

- *They don't satisfy like real food.* Let's face it, do you really want to slurp down a "shake" made from mixing some kind of powder in water or milk? Or would you rather eat a nice sandwich piled high, followed by a crunchy apple? Real foods give you not only nutrition but also the enjoyment of tasting and chewing and feeling that comfortable fullness deep in your belly. No powder can hold a candle to that.

- *It's impossible for them to contain all the nutrients of real food.* A really good artificial food may indeed contain a number of important nutrients, but there's no way it can include every good thing a real food does. For instance, many synthetic foods focus on the major nutrients such as protein and carbohydrates but leave out some of the trace elements, such as copper or selenium. In fact, scientists are continually discovering that more and more elements and compounds found in real food are important. Until this knowledge is complete, no imitation food can possibly include all the natural ingredients found in the real thing. Until scientists can create a fake steak that has not only the protein of steak but also the look, taste, and texture, you're better off sticking with the real thing when possible.

- *They may prove useful as supplements, but not food replacements.* We don't mean to imply that artificial foods are all bad or have no place in your menu. For instance, some people have trouble eating real food due to disease or injury—for them, fake foods are a lifesaver. Others have trouble eating enough food, so powders and drinks used as dietary supplements can help them get the nutrition they require. Also, we're not ruling out so-called functional foods, which fortify foods with additional nutrients such as calcium in order to yield a specific health enhancement. But don't use the imitations to replace all real food unless you can't handle the real deal.

The Risks From Relying on Artificial Foods

- *Malnutrition.* Most artificial edibles are unbalanced in one way or another. And if you rely on unbalanced food long enough, you may suffer from some degree of malnutrition. You may sustain one of the following problems.

- *Disease.* There are many documented cases of people relying on fake foods for so long that they became seriously ill.

Some have even died. Back in the 1980s, for instance, there were some very low-calorie powders with unbalanced protein. People who relied too much on them sometimes developed heart problems because their hearts weren't getting the nutrition they needed. Several dozen died from "starving their hearts." More recent formulations aren't so bad, but you still might get ill from eating them too much, to the exclusion of real and wholesome food.

- *Mood effects.* Odds are that long-term reliance on the fake stuff will make you feel bad. You'll likely feel deprived and get more tense and irritable. You may feel depressed, or weak and lethargic. Why put yourself through this? Eat some fresh fruit and vegetables and you'll feel better.

- *Long-term weight gain.* Yes, you read that right. These ads promise weight loss, and you probably will lose in the short run. But in the long term, you may actually gain more weight. After a few meals or days on the imitation junk, you will increasingly crave real food. You'll either start cheating on your diet or chuck it altogether and pig out on all the treats you've been denying yourself. Odds are, you'll gain back the lost weight and often a pound or two more! This holds true for unbalanced fad diets in general, not just those relying on fake food.

Choose Whole, Fresh Foods Instead

If your goal is to lose weight, you don't have to spend your hard-earned money on artificial powders and such anyway. Instead, concentrate on real foods that are both nutritionally sound and low in fat. Keep reading the next few chapters for more information on how to select whole, fresh foods for a balanced diet. You'll feel better as a result. You'll look better, too. And you'll slow your biological clock.

CHAPTER 10

Eat More Roots and Shoots

Studies comparing vegetarians to the rest of us have long revealed some astounding differences. People with a high intake of plant foods:

- Have lower blood pressure.
- Have less cancer and heart disease.
- Have better blood sugar balance and less diabetes.
- Are thinner and feel better.
- Live longer.

We know, you're probably thinking, "Well that's just too bad; I'm not giving up surf 'n' turf, prime rib, pork chops, and lobster. No way. Forget it. Not going to happen."

And you don't have to. More recent studies have clarified the connection. You don't have to give up all animal foods. You don't have to become a total vegetarian. You can get the great health benefits of plant foods simply by eating more vegetables and fruits (more on the latter in chapter 12). You don't have to eliminate animal foods altogether, just cut down on the amounts consumed.

Why Vegetables Are so Good for You

If your mom was typical, she urged you to eat all your vegetables when you were growing up. If you asked why, she probably said they were good for you. Of course she was right. Vegetables contain an enormous variety of healthy ingredients:

- *Vitamins and minerals.* Without enough of these, you can get sick and even die. Vegetables are loaded with them (while meat isn't).

- *Complex carbohydrates.* These provide the energy you need to keep going on a busy day. Meat has more fat and protein, but very little carbohydrate.

- *Antioxidants.* These fight cancer and aging in general. Some experts believe that one reason our body's cells get sluggish, less efficient, and just plain older is because they're constantly attacked by chemical by-products called free radicals. These brutes act like marauding savages slashing and burning their way through your cells, while antioxidants are the cavalry coming to the rescue, blasting free radicals right back into harmless chemicals again.

- *Other phytochemicals.* These chemicals provide much of the color in veggies—the orange in carrots, the green in spinach—but also much of the nutrient value. Because of this, veggies with stronger colors generally are healthier than those pale, gnarly old things left at the bottom of the bin. Phytochemicals also help the body fight cancer and aging.

Vegetables With Special Properties

All vegetables are great, but some are better than others because they pack more of a nutritional wallop. They send a lot more "cavalry" into the battle for your good health.

- *Broccoli.* Just one cup of chopped broccoli provides about 90 percent of your daily vitamin A need, 200 percent of your vitamin C need, other vitamins, important minerals such as calcium and phosphorus, fiber (more on this in chapter 13), and potent cancer-fighting chemicals such as sulforaphane.

- *Dark salad greens.* Romaine lettuce, spinach, parsley, and other darker greens are far more nutritious than their lighter cousins such as iceberg lettuce. Recent research on the antioxidant carotenoids like lutein in these greens found them to be better for aging eyes even than the well-known carrot. Lutein and related compounds protect the retina from free radicals and help prevent age-related macular degeneration (ARMD).

- *Tomatoes and tomato paste.* Studies show that people who eat more tomato products have less cancer and heart attacks. People with the highest consumption have about half the heart attack risk as those with the least! They also have far fewer cancers, according to Harvard Medical School's Dr. Edward Giovannucci, who reviewed seventy-two previous studies linking tomatoes to cancer prevention. We think one of the main reasons for this dramatic health effect is the lycopene (an antioxidant) found in tomatoes and tomato sauce.

Singling out these few vegetables does not mean we should ignore the rest. *All* vegetables are good for you.

Veggie Recipes to Make Your Taste Buds Tingle

A Word on Preparation

Cooking destroys some of the vitamins in vegetables, so eat them raw when practicable, as in salad. If you need to cook them, try steaming rather than boiling, and you'll lose 50 percent less of the nutrition. Slicing vegetables thinly exposes more of the flesh to the air, which also kills some of the nutrients. Better to slice thick, and to do so just before serving.

Don't forget vegetable juices! Most are tasty as is, but you can always add a little zing with a splash of lemon juice, a dash of hot sauce, or a sprinkle of paprika or garlic powder. Canned and bottled veggie juices are usually fine, but make sure you buy 100 percent real juice—and avoid those too high in added salt. If you're so inclined, buy a juicer and make your own.

Cold Veggie Recipes

For this and the next several chapters on good things to emphasize in your diet, we want to make sure you get started right with some delicious recipes. If you think of *vegetables* as a pile of bitter brussels sprouts or mushy overcooked cauliflower, that's not too appetizing. We want to introduce you to vegetables (and other plant foods in the next few chapters) that you can relish.

Let's start with some you can serve cold.

Vegetarian Tacos

4 taco shells
1 can vegetarian chili or cooked beans
6 ounces Cheddar cheese, shredded
4 ounces mild green chile peppers, seeded and chopped
6 ounces romaine lettuce or other greens
6 ounces taco sauce (mild or hot, according to taste)

Fill each taco shell with a bountiful serving of the chili, Cheddar, peppers, greens, and sauce. Makes 2 servings. Enjoy!

Zippy Party Dip

1 sweet pepper, chopped fine
3 jalapeño (or other hot) peppers, chopped fine
1 onion, chopped fine
8 ounces light (low-fat) sour cream

Mix thoroughly and serve with fresh vegetables such as carrot and celery sticks, cauliflower and broccoli florets, and mushroom and cucumber slices.

Hot Veggie Recipes

Some like it hot!

Vegetarian Pasta

¼ cup chopped green pepper
¼ cup chopped onion
¼ cup chopped tomato
¼ cup sliced mushrooms
1 cup cubed tofu
½ teaspoon basil
¼ teaspoon oregano
½ teaspoon salt
2 tablespoons olive oil
6 ounces spaghetti (or other pasta), cooked

Sauté the vegetables with the tofu, basil, oregano, and salt in olive oil for 5 minutes. Add the pasta and toss gently. Makes 2 servings.

Veggie Bake

1 potato, grated
1 large carrot, grated
1 zucchini or yellow squash, grated
1 cup rice, boiled and drained

Mix all the ingredients together thoroughly and spoon into a greased baking pan, smoothing into one layer. Bake at 375 degrees for 15 to 20 minutes, or until it starts to brown. Remove from the oven, let cool, and cut into squares. Makes 2 servings.

Zesty recipes such as these should make your vegetable intake more fun as well as healthful.

CHAPTER 11

Learn to Love Legumes

Legumes—beans and peas of all sorts—come close to being the ideal food. They're high in proteins useful for building muscle and a host of enzymes and other bodily chemicals, including those that help store memories. Legumes are also high in carbohydrates, valuable for providing the energy required to keep you going. They have more vitamins and minerals than many other foods and also a high degree of fiber to help keep you regular. Yet they're low in calories and fat, without a trace of cholesterol. They make a cheap and nutritious substitute for meat, which is too prevalent in many American diets. All these factors make legumes great health enhancers. A study at Tulane University found that people who eat legumes at least four times a week had a 19 percent lower chance of heart disease compared to those who ate them on average less than once a week.

The Glycemic Index

Where legumes stand head and shoulders above other carbohydrate foods is in their glycemic index (GI). The GI is a scale for ranking how quickly carbohydrate foods are broken down by the body into blood sugar. A high-GI food (such as potatoes or white bread or sugary foods—see chapter 17 for details) provides you a relatively quick surge of energy, but it disappears rapidly. That leaves you feeling hungrier and weaker than before.

But legumes are just the opposite—they release energy into the system slowly, reaching less of an intense peak than sugar, but then keeping you on a comfortable plateau far longer. Some legumes, such as lentils, have a GI that's four to five times better than that of sugar. This means that a meal rich in legumes will help keep your energy level up for hours longer than many other types of meals. This also helps you control snack cravings. If you're going to be in a situation where you can't eat for an extended period, perhaps in a long business meeting, legumes can give you the edge. After a few hours, you may note others in the meeting looking distracted, tired, or hungry while you still feel more alert and energetic.

Legumes and Gas

All these many benefits come with one major drawback: legumes are among the gassiest foods known. This is because they contain several kinds of highly complex carbohydrates, some of which your body won't fully digest. What you can't handle gets consumed in your intestines by a horde of voracious bacteria. These in turn produce copious quantities of gas, which can be both uncomfortable if you try to hold it and quite noticeable if you don't.

Luckily, there are several ways to attack this problem:

- *Find a less gassy legume.* Different people find different legumes more gassy than others. On a weekend or other convenient time, experiment with various ones to find those that affect you the least.

- *Recook beans.* Mexican chefs long ago hit on this technique as a solution. They cook, mash, and refry the beans. The extra cooking helps break down chemical bonds to make the bean starches more digestible to you . . . before they reach the gut bacteria. Unfortunately, Mexican chefs often add a lot of lard or other fat to the beans during this process. Here's a fat-free alternative: Rinse the lentils or other dry legumes, then soak them in clean water for one hour. Discard that water, add fresh water, and then boil in an uncovered pot vigorously for three minutes. Let it stand for one hour and then discard the water yet again. Add new water to about two inches above the lentils. Boil and then simmer for forty minutes. This may not stop the gas problem altogether, but it should drastically reduce it.

- *Enzyme supplements.* In recent years, scientists have found ways to provide in pill or droplet form the extra enzymes humans need to fully digest beans. Grocery stores, health food stores, and drugstores often carry such products. You just take one or two such pills or a few drops with your legumes. Then you can be sure of no bean-related gas from that meal, provided that you take enough enzyme to handle the amount of beans you're eating.

Some Tasty Legume Recipes

Each of the recipes below mentions one kind of bean, but you can try other types for variety. Canned soybeans or lentils are best if you want a very low-glycemic-index food. In fact, if you don't feel like preparing something more fancy, you can eat lentil soup or other legumes right out of the can. Just heat in a pan or microwave bowl and add seasonings to taste.

El Zippo Beans

2 15-ounce cans navy beans, drained
¾ cup water
1 8-ounce can tomato sauce
1 medium onion, chopped
1 medium apple, finely chopped
1 tablespoon mustard
1½ teaspoons Worcestershire sauce (or any hot sauce, as desired)
⅛ teaspoon pepper

Combine all the ingredients in a saucepan. Bring to a boil, then reduce the heat and cover. Cook gently for 30 minutes. Remove the cover and continue cooking for 10 minutes more.

Makes 4 servings.

Lentil Chili

1 pound dry lentils
1 teaspoon salt
5 cups boiling water
1 16-ounce can tomatoes or tomato sauce
1½ tablespoons chili powder
1 medium onion, chopped
½ cup chopped celery
1 garlic clove, minced
hot pepper to taste (optional)

Rinse the lentils, discarding any stems or stones. Add the salt and lentils to the boiling water, cover, and simmer for 30 minutes. Add the tomatoes, chili powder, onion, celery, garlic, and hot pepper (if you like). Cover and simmer for 30 minutes more.

This is best served over rice or spaghetti. Makes 7 servings.

Bean Casserole

1 cup dry lentils or other legumes, cooked
½ cup chopped walnuts
1 egg
½ cup evaporated skim milk
½ cup bread crumbs (or sugarless cornflakes)
1 large onion, chopped
1 teaspoon cumin
¼ teaspoon thyme

Mix all ingredients together thoroughly in a large bowl. Place the mixture in a greased 9 × 5 × 3–inch loaf pan and bake at 350 degrees for 30 minutes. Let cool, then serve with tomato sauce. Makes 6 servings.

A healthy serving of these or similar legume dishes will keep your energy level up for many hours, making you feel younger and more alive!

CHAPTER 12

Be Fruitful and Multiply Your Years

As we saw in chapter 7 on sugar, most of us have a strong "sweet tooth." Some of us must have more than one, for in the course of a year, we can eat our own body weight in sugar. But instead of relying on sweetened foods, do you recall the healthier alternative—the kind of natural food that already contains, in its original, unprocessed state, plenty of wholesome sweetness?

If you answered "fruit," go to the head of the class!

The Benefits of Eating Fruit

Fruit makes an ideal dessert or snack not only because it tastes sweet but also because:

- Fruit's carbohydrates energize you.

- Fruit contains lots of fiber (also see chapter 13).

- Fruit is rich with healthful vitamins.

- Fruit contains many other invaluable nutrients. For instance, citrus fruits contain chemicals such as monoterpenes that fight cancer. Many berries such as strawberries contain another anticancer compound known as ellagic acid. Blueberries are loaded with nutrients. Dried blueberries (but not fresh or frozen) are even good for relieving diarrhea. The flavonoids in colorful berries and other fruits may even relieve arthritis pain by helping reduce the swelling in arthritic joints.

- Fruit juice helps you meet your fluid requirements (see chapter 19).

- Fresh fruit is far lower in fat and calories than typical processed desserts.

- Diets high in fruit (as well as other plant foods such as vegetables) have been demonstrated to enhance health by lowering blood pressure and reducing the risk of heart disease and cancer. For instance, a study of twenty thousand middle-aged and elderly adults conducted by the University of Cambridge (England) and reported in 2001 found that eating just one more serving per day of a vitamin-C-rich fruit or vegetable reduced by 20 percent your risk of dying. This doesn't mean that popping vitamin C pills would have that much effect, because the plant foods involved contain so many more healthy nutrients in addition to vitamin C.

Over the Rainbow

Fruit Selection

Fruit comes in every color of the rainbow, from the apple's red and banana's yellow to the blue and purple of berries, the green of grapes, and the orange of citrus. As you choose fruit for your diet (at least two to four servings a day), sample from that entire spectrum of color.

In other words, don't just eat one or two kinds of fruit over and over again endlessly. That's better than eating no fruit at all, but to derive maximum benefit from this category, try to cover a large number of different fruits over a period of, say, a week or two. That way you'll get the best possible mix of fruit's benefits, since one may specialize in vitamin C, another in soluble fiber, and still another in various antioxidants.

And don't forget to sample the different varieties of the same item. For instance, there are several types of apples, from Red or Golden Delicious to McIntosh and Grannies. Pink and white grapefruit both have about the same amount of vitamin C, but the pink type has more of those color-related phytochemicals (see chapter 10) so useful in fighting disease, including twenty-five times the beta-carotene. Similarly, cantaloupe has more beta-carotene than the lighter-colored melons.

Natural or Processed

Processing destroys some of fruit's nutrients. So you'll get more benefit from a whole apple or fresh blueberries than from apple pie or blueberry cobbler. Plus the processed dessert items add tons of unnecessary sugar and fat to your diet. If you enjoy them, do so only occasionally, and count these items as optional treats rather than as fulfilling your fruit needs.

Whole Fruit or Juice?

Orange, apple, and other fruit juices taste terrific, help meet your fluid needs, and contain many of the nutrients found in whole, fresh fruit. Juice does lack some of fruit's good stuff, however, including much of the fiber. (Even juice with pulp included lacks most of the fiber found in the original fruit.) Therefore, get no more than half of your fruit servings as juice. Let at least half be whole, fresh fruit. Furthermore, when buying juice for this purpose of meeting fruit intake needs, make sure you get 100 percent real juice. Avoid the various fruit "drinks" or "ades"—which often contain only 10 percent or less of real juice (check the label to be sure). A final note on juice—fresh, unpasteurized juice sometimes contains dangerous bacteria, so only buy from reputable sources and don't store it at room temperature, which bacteria love.

Try These Great Fruit Recipes

Fresh Fruit

Don't forget to grab a whole apple, pear, orange, or the like sometimes. But do wash the peel thoroughly before you eat the fruit. Remember, that peel has probably been handled multiple times and may have pesticide residues on it. Also, wash the outside of a melon (such as a cantaloupe or honeydew melon) before cutting it open, or else the knife may carry soil and other contaminants from the outside into the edible part.

Fruit salad

Slice some apples into 8 or 16 pieces each. Add sections from citrus fruits such as oranges, some melon balls or chunks, and some grapes or raisins. Sprinkle with grated coconut and/or unsalted nuts.

Berries and Yogurt

In the days before concern over dietary fat, people would recommend berries and cream. Try skipping the cream and add a dollop of plain yogurt to a cup of fresh strawberries, blueberries, raspberries, or other desired berry.

Fruit Milk Shake

3 cups ripe fresh peaches, strawberries, or other fresh fruit
½ cup nonfat dry milk powder
1 cup water
8 ice cubes, crushed

Wash and peel the fresh fruit, if necessary. Cut it into pieces, and mash through a strainer or with a fork. Use a blender (if you have one) or beat together the fruit, milk powder, and water. Add the crushed ice and mix again.

Makes 4 servings.

Being fruitful in your diet not only adds to your dining pleasure but can also add to the years of your life—and the life of your years. Don't forget the fruit!

CHAPTER 13

Become a Fiber Fanatic

M any people suffer from chronic constipation, irritable bowel
syndrome, painful intestinal cramps, and related symptoms.
Yet they calmly continue to avoid dietary fiber, not having a clue
that they're ignoring nature's own simple remedy for all these
problems.

The Amazing Benefits of Dietary Fiber

Both soluble and insoluble dietary fiber are essential for keeping you younger and healthier:

- *Intestinal function.* Insoluble fiber in the diet absorbs water
  and expands, keeping the stool moist and giving it bulk for
  easy elimination. This prevents your system from alternating
  between the unpleasant extremes of constipation and diarrhea.

- *Cancer prevention.* Keeping the system regular helps prevent serious, life-threatening diseases as well as discomfort.

- *Heart disease.* Soluble fiber—such as that found in oats and apples, for instance—helps clear bad cholesterol from the circulatory system, lowering the risk of heart disease.

If you want to feel better every day as well as reduce the risk of deadly diseases, make sure you get plenty of fiber.

Where to Find Fiber in Food

Animal foods such as meat, fish, poultry, cheese, milk, and eggs don't provide fiber. You've got to turn to the plant kingdom to get it, though even here, many people tend to avoid fiber. For instance, white flour is what's left after most of the fiber has been removed. Whole-wheat bread and pasta, on the other hand, do provide plenty of this valuable food ingredient. Similarly, fruit juice contains much less fiber than whole fruit. Legumes such as beans, lentils, and peas are especially rich in fiber, as discussed in chapter 11.

To counteract the typical lack of dietary fiber, some processed foods like bran muffins add it, but they usually do so along with too much fat and/or sugar.

The best way to verify good fiber content is the "crunch" test. Not much crunch in a mouthful of juice, moist rice, or cooked pasta, right? Therefore, not much fiber. Now, how much crunch do you find in a whole apple, a raw carrot, or a stick of celery? Plenty, right? Therefore, plenty of fiber. The crunch test doesn't work so well with processed foods like potato chips specifically engineered to give you a crunch, however.

Enjoy These Fiber-Rich Recipes

Aim for at least one high-fiber food with each meal, and you should be okay. If this represents a major increase over your usual intake, your system may require a few days to adjust, so you should probably increase slowly.

Breakfast Cereal

Ignore the highly refined, sugary, kiddie cereals. Most of the fiber has been removed from them. Go for one of the more natural cereals—the kind that feature whole grain, or a variety of mixed grains, or some fruit chunks or nuts; their names usually brag about containing fiber. Alternatively, eat any other cereal you like, but sprinkle some bran buds, bran flakes, or other pure bran cereal on top.

Lunch

Try any of these suggestions (not necessarily all in the same meal):

- Your usual sandwich, but made with whole-wheat bread rather than white.

- Any kind of homemade soup that contains lots of different vegetables—vegetable soup, black bean soup, lentil soup, barley soup, beef and vegetable soup, minestrone soup, and so on.

- Salad—any kind with fruit and/or vegetables. But for purposes of fiber, minimize pasta salad, tuna salad, egg salad, and the like.

Snack

- Fruit—any whole piece of fruit, especially one with a crunch like an apple.

- Vegetables—try carrot and celery sticks, or broccoli and cauliflower florets, or any other veggies with a satisfying fresh crunch.

- Popcorn—few snacks have more fiber than popcorn. If you're craving something salty and crunchy, choose popcorn over the various types of processed chips.

Dinner

Bean-Green Casserole

1 cup lentils, rinsed (for variety, use any dry bean or pea)
2 cups of water
2 teaspoons mustard seeds
1 cup chopped onion
2 tablespoons olive oil
2 tablespoons cider vinegar
8 cups fresh spinach leaves, washed (for variety, use any vegetable greens)

In a medium saucepan, bring the lentils, water, and mustard seeds to a boil. Reduce the heat, cover, and simmer until the lentils are tender, about 15 minutes. Drain.

In a large skillet sauté onion in olive oil until tender, about 5 minutes. Stir in the vinegar. Add the lentils to skillet and mix thoroughly. Add the spinach, tossing until it begins to wilt. Serve warm. Makes 4 servings.

Curried Rice-Bean Delight

3 cups brown or wild rice, cooked
1½ cups red kidney beans, cooked
4 green onions, chopped
½ green pepper, diced
2 stalks celery, diced
¼ cup fresh parsley, chopped
¼ cup low-fat mayonnaise
¼ cup plain low-fat yogurt
2 teaspoons curry powder
dash of black pepper
hot pepper to taste

Combine the first six ingredients by tossing in a mixing bowl. In a separate bowl, combine the mayonnaise, yogurt, curry powder, and peppers. Then blend this mixture thoroughly with the vegetables. Serve warm or cold.

Makes 6 servings.

Mouthwatering recipes like these make getting your daily fiber fun as well as healthy!

Spice Away Disease

Spice can be very nice! It adds nuances of flavor that can transform an ordinary dish into a gourmet's paradise. Its many combinations can add infinite variety to our menus so that we need never suffer jaded taste buds. And increasingly, medical science is discovering that various spices can positively boost health.

Spices to Enhance Food Safety

All of us have experienced the angry intestinal cramps and diarrhea that result from eating tainted food and beverages. Millions suffer every year. The bigger and more severe outbreaks where hundreds get sick and some die even make the news. The best ways to avoid such problems include sanitary food handling and proper cooking. But for added insurance, take a tip from a team of microbiologists at Kansas State University who found that five common spices can kill the bacteria that frequently poison food. And guess what? These five are also among our most flavorful and delightful in the kitchen. They are garlic and cloves first of all, then—somewhat less effective—cinnamon, oregano, and sage.

Adding one or more of these spices while you're preparing a

dish like meat loaf, for example, will help keep that food fresh by suppressing bacterial growth. Once a food has become tainted, however, the damage is done, and adding spices at this point will not reverse the process.

Spices to Beat Congestion and Colds

Not too long ago, Americans associated chile peppers primarily with ethnic cooking, particularly Mexican, Szechuan Chinese, and other notoriously hot fare. Increasingly, chiles are finding their way into the mainstream, and are often found in such places as salad bars and fast-food joints. And with good reason. Not only do chiles pack a powerful taste wallop, transforming almost any dish into a fiery delight, but they also help fight respiratory ailments. The next time you feel a little congestion or a cold coming on, help yourself to some of nature's nutritional fire. Not only will your taste buds feel the tingle, but your nasal passages and sinuses will start to open up. The mucous glands will begin to run freer, your eyes will water, your nose will sniffle, and your forehead may break out in sweat. As your sinuses drain, notice how much more freely you breathe. Since congestion leads to colds or sinus infections by providing an ideal environment for bacteria to thrive, anything that breaks this cycle helps keep you healthier. Moreover, chiles are rich in fiber, vitamins A and C, and phytochemicals such as quercetin that reduce cancer risk. Perhaps best of all, we now know that the old belief that spicy foods upset your stomach and cause ulcers is only a myth. Chiles are perfectly safe for most people! (An exception: if you have food allergies, eating spicy food makes it easier for the allergens to enter your digestive system and flare up your allergic responses.)

Spices for Other Diseases

Scientists used to believe that garlic could help your heart and arteries by fighting bad cholesterol. Recent, more carefully designed studies have cast doubts on this conclusion. Nevertheless, there is a wealth of evidence that garlic may be beneficial in other ways. Garlic seems to boost the immune system, improve blood pressure, help with diabetes, and reduce the risk of cancer. It (as well as onions) may even help reduce the pain of arthritis by absorbing the toxins that irritate inflamed joints. It seems too good to be true, but the only real drawback to garlic ingestion is the powerful odor it can give your breath. There are ways around this, however. Cooking garlic helps (see recipe below), as does taking special over-the-counter breath saving pills. Another alternative is to take pills of purified garlic rather than eating it as a spice. This last idea, however, does take all the fun out of consuming garlic, and it may not be as effective as natural garlic.

Spicy Recipes for Fighting Disease

Russian Garlic Salad

50–75 garlic cloves, peeled
½ teaspoon salt
½ cup balsamic vinegar
1 cup extra-virgin olive oil
1 teaspoon freshly ground black pepper
1 tablespoon oregano

Fill a saucepan large enough to hold all the garlic with water, and bring it to a boil. When the water boils, turn off the heat and drop the garlic cloves into the hot water. Let the garlic sit in the hot water for 3 to 5 minutes. If you like your garlic strong, choose 3 minutes. The longer it stews, the mellower the garlic.

Remove the garlic from the hot water, rinse it in cold water to stop the cooking process, and place it in a large, sealable bowl.

In another bowl, dissolve the salt into the vinegar. Add the olive oil, pepper, and oregano and whisk together to make a vinaigrette. Pour over the garlic, seal, and refrigerate for at least 1 week. Serve cold. Makes 12 servings.

Hot Spicy Fish

1 tomato, peeled and diced
2 garlic cloves, diced
1 onion, peeled and diced
½ teaspoon cumin
salt to taste
2 jalapeños (or other chile peppers), chopped
splash of olive oil
1 pound cod or any other firm fish fillets
splash of lemon juice

In a dish, mix the tomato, garlic, onion, cumin, salt, and chiles. Place the mixture in a pan with a little olive oil and cook for about 5 minutes, until reduced somewhat.

Add the fish pieces on top of the sauce, sprinkle with lemon juice, and cook until fish is cooked but still firm. Serve hot over a bed of rice or pasta. Makes 4 servings.

CHAPTER 15

Supplement Your Meals

If you're like most Americans, chances are you eat a lot of your meals on the fly. In the morning, you're rushing off to work with barely seconds to throw something together and gobble it down. Midday you may be too busy to sit down for a regular meal. Instead, you grab a bite here and a snack there and a sip somewhere in between as you dash from the phone to a meeting to greeting a customer at the door. Even at dinnertime, family members may be coming and going with diverse commitments, unable to sit together for a relaxed meal and social time.

Into this mix throw hastily prepared food, junk food snacks, and fatty fast food and you've got the recipe for not only heartburn but maybe some malnutrition as well.

Common Shortages in Modern Diets

People hear the word *malnutrition* and think of starving, listless babies from some foreign country seen on TV. That is, of course, the worst form of malnutrition. But any long-term dietary imbalance with a chronic shortage in one or more key nutrients could produce some negative health consequences. Poor diet can make you feel run down, apathetic, and even ill. And surveys show that a large proportion of Americans have at least one dietary insufficiency. In more extreme cases, you can experience severe health consequences like these:

- *Lack of iron.* Too little iron in the diet reduces the supply of red blood cells, those cool little carriers of required oxygen and energy to the bodily cells. As a result, you experience anemia, lack of energy and motivation, and chronic fatigue.

- *Lack of calcium.* Without enough dietary calcium (or the vitamin D required for it to work), your bones may lack the mineral buildup they need. It will be easier for you to suffer a broken bone, and the break will be slower to heal when that happens. With advancing age, you may experience osteoporosis, or thinning of the bones. This dreaded condition—far too common in America, especially among older women—can ruin posture, lead to increased risk of severe fractures, and ultimately cut life short due to fracture-related complications.

- *Insufficient vitamin A.* This impairs night vision and can make nighttime driving riskier.

- *Low vitamin C, E, and other immune boosters.* These deficiencies increase cancer and other disease risk by diminishing the body's resistance.

Doesn't it make sense to avoid problems like these through better nutrition? This is particularly important for people with special nutritional needs. For instance, runners put a lot of stress on their skeletal structure and will need even more calcium than will those living more sedentary lives.

Ensure Dietary Balance

In chapter 5, we talked about preparing a balanced menu plan, but what happens when you just don't have the time or opportunity, as when traveling?

Take Supplements

Some experts recommend having a whole shelf full of nutritional potions, pills, and powders. We think that's too complicated. You don't have to buy out a health food store and add every nutrient singly, spoon by spoon, swallow by swallow.

We recommend taking a daily multivitamin, multimineral supplement. Get one that includes, for example, about 1,000 to 1,200 mg of calcium, 400 IU (international units) of vitamin D, 400 IU of vitamin E, and 400 mcg of folate (or folacin), as well as a variety of trace elements and compounds such as selenium and lutein. A pill like this should cover almost all your basic needs, in combination with a reasonable diet. And it's a lot easier to remember just one pill a day. If you can't find all those key nutrients in a single pill, however, you might need to add another single-nutrient pill, perhaps vitamin E. In addition, if blood tests or other medical tests taken during your annual checkups should reveal a specific deficiency—say, calcium or iron—then you might want to take a special unitary supplement such as calcium pills in addition to the multivitamin, multimineral supplement. By the way, if you haven't had a thorough medical checkup in several years, by all means get one soon. Some conditions are easily treatable if caught early, while if not discovered until much later can be more serious—even deadly.

Watch Out for Supplement Excess

One reason you shouldn't be mixing and matching too many supplementary products is the danger of excess. Too much can be just as risky as too little. For the same reason, don't take more than the recommended dose as explained on the label of your supplement, usually one a day. Don't think that if one is good, two are better. They're not!

For instance, excessive vitamin A intake (some people are more sensitive than others and reach this point more easily) can cause aches and pains, and in extreme cases has been known to kill. Excessive vitamin D can also kill. Other nutrient overabundances may not be lethal but can cause painful and debilitating diseases. For example, people taking vitamin B_6 in doses about a hundred or more times normal sometimes develop painful and disruptive nerve impairments. Better to have no supplements than a lavish surplus.

Pick the Best Supplement for You

Take a few minutes glancing over the vitamin shelf at your local pharmacy, grocery, or health food store. Note the products targeted at people your age and gender. For instance, women who are still in the childbearing years generally need more iron than do other women or men. Once you've narrowed your choice down to a handful, look on the labels to see how many different vitamins and minerals are covered. Generally, it's best to pick the supplement that offers the largest variety of vitamins and minerals. Then note on the label what percent of Daily Value (recommended daily consumption) for each nutrient is provided by a single pill. The acceptable range in most cases is about 20 percent to 100 percent. Up to about 150 percent for certain nutrients, such as vitamins C and E, may be okay. But avoid doses in the several hundred or thousand percent. This means a single pill is giving you several times the recommended daily dose—not even counting what you also get through food and beverages.

Strike a happy balance between inadequate and excessive nutrient intake, and your body will thank you for it. You may well prevent or reverse aches, pains, weakness, or lethargy that you thought was due to age but is actually under your control.

CHAPTER 16

Build Up Your Bones

Without bones, we'd be little more than long jellyfish. It is hard, rigid bone that provides structure and shape to our bodies, that allows us to walk upright, that allows movement as we know it at all. Muscles attach with tendons to our bones. When we flex our muscles, that moves our bony limbs so that we can walk, and grasp, and carry.

As important as our bones are, you'd think we'd pay a lot of attention to them and take great care of them. But we don't. Most of us take them for granted until something happens—a bone spur, a break, or perhaps osteoporosis. But by then it may be too late to do much to ensure future bone health.

Osteoporosis

As we grow older, our bones begin to gradually lose the mineral deposits that keep them strong. They become thinner, more porous, and more likely to break.

Fractures From Osteoporosis

Surely you've noticed that many older people break their hips. This causes not only pain and costly medical treatment, but also an impaired lifestyle (perhaps with loss of independence) and the risk of life-shortening complication. Experts used to think that the elderly lost their balance more with age, were thus more likely to fall, and then often broke their hips as a result. But that's not the way it usually works. How many young people, when they fall, break a hip? What's often really happening is that the elderly get such porous bones that a sudden jolt such as stepping off a curb snaps their hip, and then they fall. In other words, the bone break causes the fall, rather than vice versa.

Posture Changes From Osteoporosis

Even in the absence of dramatic breaks, osteoporosis can cause dreadful bone changes. Some elderly people get stooped over and even develop so-called dowager's humps as their backbones begin to cave in. Once this process occurs, little can be done to reverse it. Prevention is everything.

Maximize Lifelong Bone Health

The earlier you start protecting your bones, the better. Some studies indicate that what you do at age forty or fifty isn't as important as what you did for your bones in your teenage years. This shouldn't imply that after twenty, you need do nothing. You should always take care of your bones. It's just that the growing years are a much more important time in which to do this.

Nutrition and Bone Health

When your bones were rapidly growing in adolescence, did you build them strong with the finest nutritional materials available, or did you eat mostly crud and let your bones form weakly? Here are the nutrients to focus on especially when you're still growing, but also when you're older to help keep bones strong:

- *Calcium.* This is the primary building block in your bones. Rich sources include dairy (milk, cheese, yogurt), sardines, and certain green vegetables such as broccoli and spinach. A multivitamin, multimineral supplement with calcium is recommended to ensure you get at least 1,000 to 1,200 mg a day.

- *Vitamin D.* This vitamin is absolutely essential for your body to store calcium as it should and to absorb phosphorus. For this reason, milk often comes with vitamin D added. Multivitamin supplements always include it as well. Sunlight exposure (as little as ten minutes a day) stimulates the body to produce it. Other dietary sources include egg yolks, oily fish, and vegetables.

- *Phosphorus.* Too much phosphorus is bad; it can interfere with calcium absorption and deposition. Thus, you should avoid drinking too much cola and other sodas, because they contain phosphoric acid. Stick to three cans a week or less if you can bear it. The Harvard University School of Public Health conducted a study of highly active teenage girls and found that those who regularly drank carbonated colas were five times as likely to suffer a broken bone as those who drank none. Plain water, pure fruit juice, and milk are much better for you. While excess phosphorus is bad for bones, too little is also negative. You definitely need some. Rich natural sources include meat and fish, beans, milk, and nuts.

- *Fluoride.* Too much fluoride accelerates osteoporosis. Avoid excess. Do rinse your mouth well after using fluoride toothpaste so that you don't swallow much. Don't swallow fluoride rinses, either. You want fluoride only to make contact with your teeth, not to enter your whole system.

Remember to take sufficient quantities of these nutrients throughout life. A study at the Human Nutrition Research Center on Aging at Tufts University found that healthy adults over the age of sixty-five who stopped taking calcium and vitamin D supplements lost the beneficial effects on their bones that were produced earlier by the supplementation.

Exercise and Bone Health

Everyone realizes that exercise strengthens muscles, but did you know it does the same for bones? In both cases, exercise provides a strain that warns the system to prepare for next time by growing stronger. A study conducted at Cambridge University on five thousand middle-aged and older adults found that jogging and other high-impact exercises done at least two hours per week reduced the risk of hip fracture by 33 percent for men and 12 percent for women. You might think that people stressing their bodies like this would risk more fractures, but the reverse was true, as long as the exercise was on a regular basis.

This is one reason why exercise is so important throughout all life. It's also a reason why people who are out of shape must build up very gradually. Neither muscles nor bones can recover quickly after exercise, especially as you grow older. You want to put a little stress on bone, but not too much. If, after a long run, you not only have sore muscles but feel an additional ache deeper within your legs, you've overdone it. Take a couple of days off from jogging and next time don't run so much.

The Effects of Hormones on Bones

Why are older women far more likely than men to suffer from osteoporosis? Because estrogen and related female hormones help maintain bone health. At menopause, women typically experience a more sudden and steeper drop in sex hormone levels than do men of the same age. The obvious solution—prescriptions for replacement hormones—isn't for everyone. While useful in the fight against osteoporosis and some other diseases (such as heart disease), replacement hormones increase the risk of other dread diseases such as cancer. Soy products, however, provide some of the protective effects of hormones for both sexes, without the side effects.

If you're concerned about this issue, consult with your physician about whether you're a good candidate for hormone supplementation or extra soy consumption. If you are and do start to take them, make sure you get regular checkups to catch early anything that might possibly go wrong.

Few things will diminish the quality of life for an older person more than weak or brittle bones. Whatever your current age, start *now* to take care of them. This is one of the most effective ways for you to bust the potential effects of age.

CHAPTER 17

Snack on Brain Food

Why do we sometimes yearn for rich and fatty ice cream, yummy cream-filled snack cakes, greasy and crunchy potato chips, smooth milk chocolate bars, or salty peanuts and cashews? One reason is suggestibility. Didn't simply reading that list of tasty treats suddenly make you salivate for some? You see someone on TV—or in your kitchen—eating it and, of course, you've got to have some, too!

Another reason is that our brains often demand the comfortable feeling provided by such delicious fare.

But if we would but feed our brains correctly in the first place, we could minimize the unpleasant imbalances that unleash these cravings. For maximum vigor and performance throughout our stress-filled days, the brain requires a steady supply of both energy and protein.

Grab the Gusto

To operate at all, your brain requires energy. And unlike many other bodily organs, it can't use just any kinds of potential fuel. Your muscles, for example, like to burn glucose (blood sugar) for fuel, but can also do a pretty good job burning protein or fat. The brain is more particular. It demands that the rest of the body continue to supply it with a generous helping of glucose or it gets cranky and irritable. Then the body will start converting other nutrients into glucose to ship to the brain. Or if you haven't eaten in a while (as during a diet), the body will even start to destroy its own tissue—typically muscle—to provide that steady supply of glucose.

Do you remember in chapter 11 on legumes when we talked about the glycemic index? Foods with a high index rush glucose to the brain, but unfortunately soon run out of steam. So the brain experiences rapid ups and downs in its fuel supply. But foods with a low glycemic index moderate that flow of glucose, keeping up a steady supply for a longer time. The brain stays alert, vigorous, and happy. It keeps cravings in check.

Here is a table of the glycemic index values of many common foods.

Glycemic Index of Various Foods

FOOD	GLYCEMIC INDEX
Low-Glycemic-Index Foods (slow energy release)	
Soybeans (canned)	20
Cherries	32
Plum	34
Grapefruit	36
Peach	40
Red lentils	43
Skim milk	46
Pear	47
Chickpeas	49
Ice cream	52
Yogurt (plain)	52
Apple	53
Kidney beans	54
Standard Comparison Food	
White bread	100

Glycemic Index of Various Foods (cont.)

FOOD	GLYCEMIC INDEX
High-Glycemic-Index Foods (rapid energy release)	
Instant potato	116
Cornflakes	119
Honey	126
Baked russet potato	135
Pure glucose	138

Adapted from: D. J. A. Jenkins, et al., "The Glycaemic Response to Carbohydrate Foods," *Lancet*, 2, no. 388 (1984).

Rather than trying to memorize this table, note that the best GI values generally come from complex carbohydrate plant foods. So just pick any of those that you like. Here's some possible examples:

Brain-Power Snacks

FRUITS	VEGETABLES	WHOLE-GRAIN ITEMS
Apple	Broccoli flowerets	Biscuit or roll
Grapes	Carrot sticks	English muffin
Melon	Cauliflower	"Lite" popcorn
Orange	Celery sticks	Pretzels
Pear	Tomato juice	Whole-wheat toast

The antioxidants (like vitamins C and E) and other vitamins in the fruits and vegetables listed here also help the brain function and slow the cognitive declines sometimes seen with aging. For instance, a study at Tufts University on men in their fifties found that those with the lowest levels of the B vitamins did the worst on cognitive and memory tasks.

Nab Your Neurotransmitters

In addition to energy, the other major nutrient that the brain specifically requires for continuous, smooth functioning is protein. It uses protein for all sorts of functions, including cellular repair, enzyme production, and memory formation. But the function we most need to emphasize now for daily performance is the production of neurotransmitters.

The brain uses a variety of neurotransmitters to send signals from one brain cell (neuron) to another. A neurotransmitter of particular importance during times of stress is norepinephrine, which is made from a component of protein known as tyrosine. Therefore, when your brain is struggling furiously to cope with your daily stress, it needs a good supply of tyrosine to keep from giving out. Here are some foods rich in tyrosine to help give you that stress-resisting boost:

Foods High in Tyrosine
(ranked in order of declining amount)

Eggs
Skim milk
Brewer's yeast
Cheese (especially Parmesan and Cheddar)
Soybeans
Peanuts
Cottage cheese
Peas
Sunflower seeds
Beef
Wheat germ
Tuna

Note that some foods, like legumes, are found on both lists. They're high both in complex carbohydrates and in tyrosine— super foods for brain power. Beware, however, of foods too high in fat, even if they do appear on these tables. Sure, you can have eggs occasionally, for example. They're great for many reasons, but do avoid excessive intake (more than about four per week).

The next time you know you're in for a long business meeting or about to join a stressful team project or something else that's draining, grab a brain-power snack first. You'll really notice the difference! You'll feel and act younger and more vigorous.

Take care of your brain, and it will take care of you.

CHAPTER 18

Take Unique Nutrients for Special Situations

Food doesn't just keep you healthy and alive. Certain foods and nutrients have distinct effects on your mind, mood, and performance. For example, in the last chapter on brain food, we touched on the effectiveness of antioxidants in maintaining brain function. It's time now to explore more fully some other fascinating connections between the nutrients we ingest and the behavioral or health effects that may result.

Performance Enhancement

Facilitating Sleep and Jet-Lag Adjustment

In traveling to his speaking engagements around the world, Charles frequently runs into the problem of jet lag, as do millions of other distance travelers every year. Sometimes, no matter how tired he is, it's tough to unwind, relax, and fall asleep. On his first flight back to the States from Tokyo, try as he might, he couldn't get a wink of sleep in almost twenty-four hours. That's a miserable experience.

Prescription or over-the-counter sleeping pills are usually not the best solution. These generally work, but they often leave a sort of hangover effect that keeps you dragging throughout the next day.

The answer in such cases may be nutritional supplements (but consult your physician first). Tryptophan, for instance, is an amino acid, one of the components of ordinary protein in the diet. If you swallow a pill of purified tryptophan about an hour before going to bed, it gets into your bloodstream, crosses into the brain, and there increases the production of a natural neurotransmitter called serotonin. This helps you fall asleep, stay asleep, and wake up without any drugged-out spaciness the next day. Alternatively, you can have a high-carbohydrate snack about an hour before retiring, perhaps plain crackers, jelly beans, or gumdrops. Such foods increase your insulin response, which tends to drive all the amino acids out of your bloodstream—except the tryptophan that's already there from your last protein-containing meal. This also increases serotonin and sleepiness. But beware of consuming warm milk or other protein-containing products just before bedtime, because the other amino acids in whole protein will interfere with this tryptophan effect.

A different approach is to ingest pills of the natural hormone melatonin, which helps regulate the sleep-wake cycle. Melatonin will not only help you sleep during the period right after you take it, but also help reset your biological rhythm. Thus, melatonin may be just the answer if you're experiencing jet lag or must change sleep-wake shifts due to work schedules or for any other reason. Note that adults with autoimmune disorders or allergies and all children should avoid taking it.

Boosting Mental Alertness

Another amino acid is tyrosine, and it has generally the opposite effects from tryptophan. It helps you resist stress and stay alert and active during periods of tension and fatigue. All normal protein foods contain it, but those listed in chapter 17 contain especially high amounts. Consider such foods for maximum alertness as well as the ability to concentrate and think clearly.

Caffeine from ordinary coffee, tea, chocolate, and certain over-the-counter pills also aids alertness when you're tired. We don't recommend using large quantities of caffeine every day, because this stimulant tends to cause insomnia and leave you more tired the next day. It can also become habit forming, requiring a regular dose just to make you feel as usual (as opposed to more pepped up than typically). For occasional or emergency use, however, it may prove very helpful if you're exhausted but must keep performing.

The herb ginkgo biloba has somewhat similar effects, enhancing memory for some, especially older people who are beginning to experience memory difficulties. Ginkgo seems to have multiple mechanisms for helping the brain, serving as an antioxidant as well as affecting blood flow and neurotransmission in the brain.

Mood Enhancement

Beating the Blues

Depression is one of the most common disorders in the world. Sometimes people use the word *depression* as a synonym for *sadness*. But in cases severe enough to be concerned about, the word implies a great deal more. Sufferers may feel lifeless and apathetic, may fail to enjoy their usual pursuits and pleasures, and may feel that life no longer has meaning, which poses possible suicide risks. In such serious cases, herbal remedies are no substitute for accredited diagnosis, psychotherapy, and other treatment. If you're basically in control but experiencing mild blue spells, however, consider trying the herb St.-John's-wort, which is now available in pill form. A lot of people suffer from various degrees of seasonal affective disorder, where the reduced period of sunlight during the winter months makes them bluer than usual. A mild degree of blues like this may respond very well to St.-John's-wort.

If your problem is light related, another possibility is to buy a bank of full-spectrum lights. These lights provide all the natural wavelengths that the sun does, rather than the reduced spectrum found with ordinary electric lights. Using them for two or more hours per day helps make up for the restricted natural light periods found during the winter, or among people who work indoors without windows all day.

Disease Resistance

Beating Colds

Your best bet for all-around disease resistance is a solid, balanced diet throughout the year. Still, it may pay to supplement your diet at times of disease exposure or when your bodily resistance is reduced due to stress and fatigue. For years, some people have sworn by vitamin C supplements. If you go this route, please avoid excess, which may risk problems such as gastric disturbance and even kidney stones. More recently reported possibilities include using zinc lozenges and the herbals echinacea and ginseng to boost disease resistance. Echinacea, for example, is a plant of the daisy family and often helps with not only bacterial but also viral and fungal infections of the upper respiratory tract. Though echinacea seems to boost immunity in the short term, some recent evidence suggests that long-term use may suppress immunity, leaving you worse off than before. This implies that the best plan is to take it only for a short period when you've been exposed to an illness such as the flu or feel the beginnings of a cold or other illness coming on.

Staying healthy and in primo mental shape are great ways to bust the effects of age and make you feel younger than your years. Why let the common problems discussed here drag you down when you can so easily resist them?

CHAPTER 19

Tank Up With Water

Your body's cells are made up of water more than anything else. The reason is that water is essential for all the bodily functions that maintain life. Absorbing nutrients requires water. So does transporting nutrients and oxygen throughout the body and bringing waste products to the kidneys. Water is also needed to facilitate the elimination of waste products from the body.

Do you take in enough fluids? Chances are you don't, at least some of the time. Very few people in modern America don't eat enough, but plenty don't drink enough.

There are many reasons for this, but the main one is that the thirst drive isn't all that accurate. By the time you feel thirsty, you're getting really dehydrated. At the point where you first start "drying out" and should drink a bit more, you don't yet feel thirst.

Hazards of Dehydration

Getting dehydrated doesn't merely make you experience the annoying discomfort of thirst. It can also have negative consequences for your immediate and long-term health. Let's look at some increasingly severe signs that can appear as dehydration worsens:

- *Mild.* General discomfort, loss of appetite, loss of motivation, some mental confusion, performance decline. At this point, there may be no conscious sense of thirst at all.

- *Moderate.* Headache, dizziness, serious mental confusion, difficulty speaking, walking, and so on.

- *Severe.* Mental delirium, loss of muscle control, kidney shutdown, ultimately death if you can't get some fluids.

- *Long-term consequences.* Just one severe episode or even moderate dehydration that's prolonged or frequently repeated over a number of years can increase the risk of certain physical problems such as kidney stones, urinary tract infections, and even cataract blindness.

The amazing thing is that you don't have to be trapped in the desert without water to experience some of these problems. Plenty of people with unlimited access to fluids slip into states like these without even realizing why!

How Much to Drink?

If you can't completely rely on your thirst drive to protect you, what can you trust? You need to follow recommended guidelines and learn how to check for physical symptoms other than thirst. The U.S. Army, for example, has a program of "water discipline" when troops are in the field. It prescribes drinking water on a fixed schedule whether the soldiers feel thirsty or not. If you're on your own, however, here are some suggestions.

Under Normal Conditions

During a regular day of work or school indoors with moderate temperature and no special physical exertion, plan on drinking at least eight glasses of water and other fluids per day. We're talking about a standard eight-ounce glass or half a pint per serving. Spread out this consumption throughout the day, making especially sure to drink some first thing in the morning.

Special Situations Requiring More

- *Temperature.* The hotter it is, the more you sweat, and the more lost fluids you need to replace. Most people don't realize that in very cold weather, you also need to drink more. Why? Because you exhale lots of body water in the form of vapor with each breath you take.

- *Exertion.* When you exercise more, you've got to drink more regardless of the weather. We remember a case at a state police training camp a few years ago in which the recruits exercised for several hours one afternoon without getting any water. Several ended up in the hospital with severe dehydration, a few near death. Just a couple of hours of exercise in normal weather, even less in extreme weather, can get you very dehydrated if you don't consume fluids. During heavy exercise you can lose two to four quarts of water per hour in sweat. (There's your eight glasses of intake for a regular day gone in just one hour.)

- *Climate.* If the air is drier (low humidity) or the altitude greater, you need to drink more.

- *Illness.* When you're sick, you need to drink more, especially if you have a fever. When ill, you generally don't feel like drinking, but failure to do so only makes you feel worse. So you have to force yourself.

- *Dry food.* Try eating a bag of popcorn without fluid. It's possible to do it, but you'll feel awful later—not only dehydrated, but probably constipated the next day as well.

The Sure Sign You've Had Enough

You've probably lost track of how many glasses to drink daily. Never fear. You can't trust thirst, but there is one bodily sign that always tells you when you've had enough: urine. If you're even slightly dehydrated, you'll produce a smaller amount of urine than you usually do, and it'll be darker. When you've been drinking enough, you'll produce a greater volume and it will be lighter and clearer. The only exception to this rule is if you've had a multivitamin pill or other medication within the last couple of hours that can turn your urine a bright yellow (or other color) regardless of how much fluid you've consumed. This effect shouldn't last long, however, and you can still judge dehydration by the volume produced.

The best approach, therefore, is to begin drinking water and other fluids shortly after arising and keep drinking periodically throughout the morning until you have to go to the bathroom. Continue to drink until you void clear urine. After a few weeks of this procedure, you should develop a feel for how much you should drink whether you feel thirsty or not.

Fluid Consumption and Weight Control

As part of your new, healthier eating plan, you don't want to consume too many calories in the beverages you drink. Lots of juice, regular soda, and sugar-sweetened drinks such as coffee, tea, Kool-Aid, and hot chocolate could easily add five hundred to a thousand calories a day to your intake.

Minimize Highly Caloric and Sweetened Beverages

When you're drinking for the purpose of consuming adequate fluid, we recommend just pure, simple water. There are no calories in cool, clear water! Of course, it's good to drink some milk and juice each day, but don't rely exclusively on such drinks to get your eight or more daily glasses of fluid. We've already suggested mini-mizing caffeine intake in coffee, tea, and soda because too much disturbs your rest cycle. Now here are two more reasons to control this intake—calories and the dehydrating effect of caffeine. (It's a diuretic, meaning that it promotes the loss of body water in excess urine.) Alcohol is also a diuretic.

What about sugar-free, low-calorie beverages? As we discussed in chapter 7, research has shown that the sweet taste of a sugar-free cola stimulates hunger and eating. In other words, you may only drink in one or two calories with your sugar-free cola or other artificially sweetened beverage, but it may increase your appetite and cause you to eat another couple of hundred calories. An occa-sional soda is okay, but we don't recommend relying upon them as your main thirst quencher.

Use Beverages to Help Control Eating

Here's a neat trick: before a meal or snack, drink a big glass of water. The sheer volume in your stomach makes you feel fuller and less likely to overeat. If the tap water in your area is no good, try bottled water or a home water purifier unit. There are different types of these, varying a bit in method of action and expense. Some require attachment to your sink faucet. Others are freestanding jugs with filters and ion exchange chemicals to soften the water.

Few things can make you seem worn out as fast as can dehydra-tion. Instead, tank up with water to maximize your mood, mental acuity, and overall sense of well-being. This is one very easy way to reduce how old you feel!

PART III

Protect Your Body

In part I we talked about shaping your body with exercise, and in part II about building your body by providing the nutrients and water it needs for health. Now we'll consider the external hazards—everything from medications to sunlight to bacterial invasion—that can harm your body and how you can protect yourself.

CHAPTER 20

Avoid Drug-Nutrient Interactions

It's kind of scary to realize that two things that may be helpful separately can, if taken together, harm or even kill you. It's true. For instance, if you take a certain kind of antidepressant, you may find it very helpful in controlling deeply sad and troubling moods. If you like aged cheese, that's fine by itself for most people. But if you mix both of the above, you're headed for trouble. The kind of antidepressant known as a monoamine oxidase inhibitor (MAOI) prevents the body from breaking down monoamines. And aged cheese, for example, is full of monoamines. The average person can break these down without difficulty, but if you've got MAOI in your system, you can't. The excess monoamines from the cheese are then free to play havoc with your blood pressure. Theoretically, they could cause a blood pressure spike severe enough to trigger a potentially fatal stroke or heart attack. So two things that individually are just fine could in combination prove serious or even deadly. Talk about a dismal way to cut short your biological clock!

The message here is, first, that all medications can have potentially unpleasant side effects, at least for some people. Second, know what you're taking and watch out for possibly dangerous combinations.

Get Advice

- *Ask your physician.* Make sure he or she knows what other drugs you are already taking so you won't be prescribed one that conflicts. Discuss any unexpected side effects you experience while taking the medication prescribed. Ask what foods you should increase or avoid while taking the medicine. For instance, some drugs are best taken on an empty stomach, while others are best on a full belly. If you reverse the way you should do it, you'll probably experience much discomfort and/or an unnecessary reduction in the drug's effectiveness.

- *Consult your pharmacist.* It's best to get all your prescription medicines at the same place so that your pharmacist has records of everything you are taking. He or she may then detect a possible bad combination that your doctor missed. If you get prescriptions from more than one doctor (say, a general practitioner and a specialist), it becomes especially important to keep your pharmacist informed as well as all your doctors.

- *Read the caution labels.* Most of the common, dangerous drug-nutrient interactions are well known to experts, and the labels will have complete information on what to avoid while taking that medication. If you're taking over-the-counter meds, it becomes increasingly important for you to stay informed on your own, because your doctor and pharmacist won't have a clue which of these you're taking unless you inform them. Most people avoid reading the tiny print on the little inserts that come in boxes of medicine. Don't make this mistake.

  We once had a friend who began to experience blurred vision and headaches. When asked by her physician, she said she wasn't taking any other medications, so he began to suspect a brain tumor and ordered all sorts of expensive tests.

When we learned of this, we asked her if she was by any chance taking over-the-counter ibuprofen. It turned out she was, and that the symptoms she was experiencing are common side effects given the dose she was taking and the amount of time she'd been doing so. She had failed to mention the ibuprofen to her doctor because she didn't consider over-the-counter items as real medicine. But they are! With more complete information, her doctor was able to handle her case better.

Avoid These Types of Drug-Nutrient Interactions

Here are some possible interactions to watch out for.

How Drugs Can Affect Nutrition

- *Drugs can affect food intake.* They can make you gain or lose appetite, affecting caloric intake, nutrient balance, and body weight. For instance, certain painkillers make some people gain a couple of pounds.

- *Drugs can affect nutrient absorption.* For instance, alcohol interferes with the body's ability to absorb key nutrients. If you drink, you'll need more of those. Cholesterol-lowering drugs reduce the absorption of such nutrients as folic acid, iron, and calcium. On the other hand, citrus juice enhances the absorption of dietary iron.

- *Drugs can interfere with nutrient metabolism.* For instance, anticonvulsant drugs for epilepsy can cause vitamin D and folic acid deficiencies. Diuretics to increase fluid loss can also lead to serious potassium depletion. Even the simple, almost universal drug aspirin can lower body levels of folic acid and increase the urinary loss of thiamin and vitamins C and K. Some drugs, like birth control pills, can simultaneously raise body levels of some nutrients (vitamin A, calcium, iron) and lower the levels of others (riboflavin, folic acid, and vitamin C).

How Nutrients Can Affect Drug Performance

- *Food can alter drug absorption.* Food may speed up or slow down absorption, thus affecting levels in the blood. Calcium from dairy products, for instance, reduces the absorption of the antibiotic tetracycline.

- *Foods can interfere with drug metabolism.* For instance, acidic fruit juices or soda can make some drugs dissolve too quickly, before they reach the intestines where they can be absorbed better.

- *Foods can counteract drugs.* For example, natural licorice (but not synthetic) can reverse the beneficial effects of blood-pressure-reducing medicine, thus raising blood pressure instead.

Other Drug-Drug or Nutrient-Nutrient Interactions

We don't want to imply in the above that it's only a matter of drugs affecting nutrients and vice versa. Sometimes two drugs combine to seriously disturb your system. For instance, many antihistamines and other medications can make you drowsy. If you add alcohol, too, the urge to sleep can become irresistible. Imagine the danger if you mixed both and tried to drive! Similarly, herbs that some people take as performance enhancers can interfere with drugs. For instance, the herb ginkgo biloba, taken by some to enhance memory, can interact with the blood thinner coumadin used to dissolve or prevent blood clots. The combination could cause serious bleeding in the event of an injury. Ginkgo interacts with aspirin the same way. The herb St.-John's-wort, often taken to beat a mild case of the blues, can make birth control pills less effective. This list is not at all comprehensive, but does suggest some of the more common problems that may arise. Still, consult your physician, pharmacist, or other health professional about any other possible combination that concerns you. For more information on possible interactions as well as other concerns about drugs, such as side effects, you can also consult the online Web site www.rxlist.com. The Food and Drug Administration (FDA) Web site is another good source for drug safety information: www.fda.gov/cder/drug.htm.

CHAPTER 21

Screen Your Medicine Cabinet

In chapter 18, we pointed out the potential benefits of all sorts of nutritional supplements and herbal concoctions. But now it's time to balance the pro side of pills with the con side. Both are important. As in so much of life, maintaining balance is critical. Too much of something can be as unhealthy or dangerous as too little.

Almost everyone is aware that illegal drugs can often kill, sometimes with a single dose. For instance, the basketball player Len Bias, right after winning a lucrative professional contract, died after his first exposure to cocaine. If even a young and vigorous athlete can be felled by a single dose of illegal drugs, imagine the risks for someone older or in lesser shape.

But does this imply that all legal drugs are perfectly safe? Emphatically, no! You should take precautions with all the over-the-counter as well as prescription medicines and with nutritional or herbal supplements or remedies you try. Here are some guidelines.

Wisely Use Medicine

- *Note expiration dates.* Just like food items, most drugs have expiration dates. Periodically screen your medicine cabinet, looking for expired dates. Each time you take a medicine, note the expiration date first. Take these dates seriously. If you can, plan to use up your older stocks first so that you don't have to waste them. But if you have some left when a medicine expires, throw it out. After expiration, some drugs lose their potency, while others chemically break down into hazardous by-products. Either way, you don't want to put this mess into your body. Don't take a chance—just get rid of it. To make sure no children get into these discarded supplies, we recommend that you *don't* just dump the whole bottlefuls and boxfuls on top of an open trash can. Actively destroy the stock in some way, perhaps flushing the pills down the toilet or running them through your garbage disposal. At the very least, seal your discards into a trash bag and remove it from the house at once, taking it to your trash disposal area.

- *Don't exceed recommended dosages.* Many drugs are available in stronger form only by prescription but can be found in weaker form over the counter. For example, the pain reliever ibuprofen may be prescribed in pills of 400 mg, 600 mg, or 800 mg each. But you can also get it without a prescription, over the counter, in the form of 200 mg pills. By gulping multiple pills, it would obviously be easy for you to get the same dose per time as found in the prescription strength. But don't do this unless recommended by a physician. Follow the directions to use the least possible dose to achieve pain relief. Your liver and kidneys dispose of most drugs in your system. But if you consume too much, you can overwhelm your system and cause organ damage.

- *Stay alert to possible side effects.* If you're under a doctor's care, he or she will be on the alert for negative side effects. If you're self-prescribing with over-the-counters, you're on your own. Read the warning insert found in most medicine boxes or on the bottle label. This will tell you when the medicine is called for and when you shouldn't take it. The label will also list the most common adverse reactions. While taking the medicine, note any new or unusual symptoms that arise. If they're serious, by all means consult your physician. If they're minor, discontinuing the drug or reducing the dose may be enough to make them go away.

- *Beware of drug interactions.* Chapter 20 covered this in much greater detail, but we want to remind you that many drugs that work quite well when given singly can have toxic or even lethal results when combined. Generally, the risk is greatest with the stronger prescription drugs, and your physician and/or pharmacist will probably warn you about possible interactions to avoid. But as mentioned earlier, always remain alert to negative side effects when taking either a single medication or a combination of them.

Popular Items to Use Cautiously or Avoid

Just because an item is labeled a "health" food or comes from a "health food" store doesn't necessarily mean it will promote health. The health food industry is less regulated by the government than either the health industry or the food industry. Some compounds that would be illegal to sell as over-the-counter medications are perfectly legal when sold as nutritional supplements. This makes no scientific or medical sense at all, but merely reflects current political and legal realities. Therefore, consumers should take special precautions when buying and using health food items for which miraculous healing abilities are claimed. Here are but a few examples; this is not a complete and exhaustive list—that would require an entire book.

Herbal Remedies

There is increasing scientific data that some herbal concoctions do have merit, as discussed in chapter 18. This does not mean, however, that every herb does all the magical things claimed for it. And there's another problem with herbs, whether consumed in whole or natural form, pill form, or as a tea. Unlike purified pharmaceutical drugs, with an herb you never know the exact dose that you're getting of the useful active ingredient(s). One time you may gobble less than you need, another time more. Furthermore, you don't know exactly what other compounds in that plant you may be exposing yourself to. Some of these may be toxic or give you allergy problems. For instance, ginseng is often taken to enhance alertness, but it also can have deleterious side effects. Ginseng may increase blood pressure and insomnia, while echinacea sometimes triggers allergies, and ginkgo biloba can cause headaches or allergies, too. Herbs such as comfrey, chaparral (in pill form), and kombucha tea can cause serious liver disease. Therefore, when using an herbal remedy, always be alert for adverse reactions.

Ergogenic Aids

These are compounds said to enhance athletic performance. Sports magazines, among others, list all sorts of supplements that promise to build muscle, boost endurance, and generally turn you into a superman. When you see incredible claims for any product, always be suspicious. Look for scientific evidence to support the claims. Most ergogenic aids are fairly expensive considering that only some of them work, and then only under certain circumstances. For instance, sodium bicarbonate helps anaerobic exercisers such as weight lifters reduce the buildup of lactic acid in their muscles, thus enabling them to work out longer. It won't, however, help aerobic exercisers like runners and ball players. But most of the claims are just hype. For instance, bee pollen and royal jelly are great for bees, but don't do much for humans. Creatine supplements may provide a slight help to elite athletes who have already reached their peak, but can worsen performance in lesser specimens by adding water weight. As the old Romans used to say, *"Caveat emptor!"*—"buyer beware."

CHAPTER 22

Protect Your Pearly Whites

It's a good thing that we get two sets of teeth in a lifetime, or an awful lot of us would be toothless by our twenties or thirties. Not many years ago, even with two sets to live on, plenty of people were wearing false teeth by middle age. Those juvenile chompers don't last long, and many people take such poor care of their one set of permanent teeth that these don't last a lifetime either. There are still far too many people who have lost teeth that could have been saved with proper care at an early enough time.

It wasn't always so. As we pointed out in chapter 7, prehistoric people in the days before refined sugar generally had better teeth at death (as revealed by their skulls discovered in the current era) than many moderns at the same age. Sugar is the prime culprit in causing tooth decay. Still, even though we live in a sugar-obsessed age, we can take better care of our teeth and make them last a lifetime. Bust this sign of age, and put off the advent of dentures as long as you can . . . hopefully forever!

Types of Dental Problems

Visualize your teeth or look in the mirror. Each tooth has a hard, bony, usually whitish outer layer called enamel. Within each tooth are living tissues called dentin and pulp, and these have blood circulation, nerves, and so on. The root of each tooth is normally securely stuck in the bone of the upper or lower jaw. The pinkish gums surround the root area and the middle portion of tooth surface so that only the uppermost portion is normally visible. Without proper dental care, you can readily experience problems with any or all parts of this system.

- *Cavities.* The bacteria that are always found in the mouth love sugar. When they get some, they use it as food and produce acids as a by-product. These acids eat away at the enamel. If you don't clean your teeth regularly, enough may be destroyed to cause a little black hole. This is much more likely if you have food—particularly sweets—stuck between teeth for an extended period. You may not detect a cavity at first, but if you allow it go untreated, the rot will eventually extend into the inner area of the tooth where the nerves are. Once the nerves get involved, you'll have a toothache. Significant, untreated tooth decay can also lead to an infection that may be not only painful but also threatening to your overall health.

- *Tooth sensitivity.* Even in the absence of tooth decay, the enamel may grow thin from such factors as excessive brushing or disease. The nerves may then lie close enough to the surface to scream out at the presence of hot, cold, sweet, or acidic foods and drinks.

- *Tooth fractures or damage.* Sometimes multiple cavities and dental repair (fillings) leave very little of the original tooth surface left. In such cases, the thin remaining wall is more likely to break if you bite down on something hard like ice cubes, jawbreaker candy, or a bit of hard bone or foreign object mixed in with your ground meat or other food. Some people also have behavioral disorders such as bruxism, or grinding of their teeth during sleep. Such problems can also wreak considerable damage on the teeth. Then there are, of course, innumerable types of falls, collisions, and other accidents that can mechanically chip or otherwise damage the teeth.

- *Gum disease.* Gingivitis and other inflammations of the gums, if untreated, can make the gums pull back from the teeth, exposing and damaging them. If they remain untreated, tooth loss can result.

Preventing Tooth Damage or Loss

Eat Right for Healthy Teeth

Just like any other part of your body, your teeth had to grow using the materials your diet made available at the time. During childhood and adolescence, teeth grow best if the diet includes sufficient protein and the key minerals calcium, phosphorus, and fluoride. Growing young people especially need multiple servings of calcium-rich foods every day. But what about when you're already grown and beginning to age? Your permanent teeth are, perhaps, decades old—what then? There's a lot of controversy now about water fluoridation, but it seems that some fluoride in the diet, in toothpaste, or in mouth rinses helps prevent cavities. There's some concern, however, that ingesting excessive amounts may be bad for the skeleton, predisposing us to osteoporosis and its consequences, such as hip fractures. So this is another area of life where a little bit of something is good for you, but a bit more can become too much.

Eating right for healthy teeth implies not only adding the right foods but also minimizing the wrong ones, most notably sugary, sweet foods. Sure, you can have a little dessert or a sweet snack now and then. You would be wise to brush your teeth thoroughly soon after, though. (Mouth bacteria begin producing acids within seconds of receiving sugar.) But what if you're at a meeting or driving or somewhere else that you can't brush? Here's a little-known trick that's very useful in cutting down on acid production following sugar consumption: the moment you finish eating the sweet or starchy food, eat something that's both nonsweet and crunchy enough to help scrub the sugar right off your teeth. Try such foods as peanuts, other unsweetened nuts, popcorn, carrot sticks, celery stalks, and broccoli spears. Though not crunchy, cheese may also help. For this purpose, avoid naturally sweet and sticky fruits such as raisins, dates, or dried apricots. This approach isn't quite as good as brushing, but it's a lot better than doing nothing. The worst thing you can possibly do is eat something sweet and let its remains sit on your teeth for hours and hours afterward. It's also rough on your chompers if you continually sip sugared beverages such as soda pop or chew sugary gum throughout the day.

Maintain Regular Dental Hygiene

Brush, if possible, after every meal or sweetened snack. If this isn't feasible, brush at least twice a day, most particularly after your last food or sweetened beverage intake of the day. Don't let sugar or other food stick to your teeth all night long.

Some people use the same toothbrush for months or even years, until the bristles look like unkempt weeds or start to fall out. Not a good approach. Worn-out bristles don't clean well, and an old toothbrush probably has a collection of old germs on it. Replace your toothbrush every two to three months at the latest. If you've just recovered from the flu or another illness, throw out the old brush regardless of its age and use a new one. Don't take a chance on reinfecting yourself.

Floss between your teeth at least once a day. Flossing can remove not only the visible particles of food stuck between teeth even after a good brushing, but also the largely invisible plaque, which is a sticky residue of bacteria on the teeth.

If you're prone to gum inflammation (reddened, swollen, tender, or painful gum areas), low doses of anti-inflammatory medications like aspirin (100 mg or so per day) may help prevent gum disease. We don't mean to suggest that aspirin can take the place of regular cleaning and professional checkups, but it may add another weapon in your overall fight for good oral health.

See Your Dentist Regularly

Most experts recommend a professional teeth cleaning twice a year and a complete exam at least once a year. If you experience dental pain or other apparent problems, see your dentist as soon as you can.

Your pearly whites can last a lifetime. Do your best to see that they do. Moreover, good oral health is an important component of your total health. Research at the State University of New York, Buffalo, discovered that an unhealthy mouth could lead to chronic obstructive pulmonary disease, a potentially fatal condition. Apparently, uncontrolled oral bacteria can lead to infections elsewhere in the body as well, in this case moving right from the mouth up into the respiratory tract.

CHAPTER 23

Shun Too Much Sun

Most of us grew up with the notion that nothing looked better than a "healthy tan." People were automatically suspicious of anyone who looked pale during the summers back in those days. Questions would arise: "Are you feeling all right?" "Why do you stay indoors all the time?" To gain the approval of our peers, many of us as teenagers deliberately baked ourselves in the sun to produce that so-called healthy glow. Then later in life, some of us developed potentially lethal forms of skin cancer. This was no coincidence.

The Deadly Hazards of Too Much Sun

Skin Cancer

Many factors play a role in the development of skin cancer, but probably the most important is excessive sun exposure, particularly sunburns. There are several types of skin cancer, but the most common are carcinoma and melanoma. Both require treatment, of course, but the former is generally not life threatening. A carcinoma typically appears as a reddish raised spot looking a bit like a volcano with an open top. It may look something like a popped pimple that doesn't heal.

Melanoma looks very different and is far more deadly. Left untreated, melanoma almost invariably kills. It's therefore essential that you get checked at the very first sign of a possible melanoma. These signs include a sudden change in a mole so that it's larger and much darker, with an irregular border. It stands up from the skin as if swollen, whereas an ordinary mole typically is closer to the same level as the surrounding skin. If you observe such a change, see your physician at once and have it removed and sent for cancer screening. Skin cancer these days is so prevalent that it accounts for about half of all cancers, according to the American Cancer Society, although most of these are the less serious carcinomas. About thirty-two thousand Americans develop malignant melanoma every year, however, and sixty-eight hundred will die.

Other Sun-Related Hazards

Not everyone who gets a lot of sun will develop cancer. But nearly all of them will prematurely age their skin. To bust this sign of age, you want to both stay healthy and look healthy. Excessive sun over a long period (even if just to the level of tanning rather than burning) tends to cause wrinkles and discolor the skin (causing so-called liver spots or age spots). People who continuously overdo sun exposure for decades when young often end up with skin that looks almost like leather. And the converse is true, too: controlled sun exposure = protected skin = looking more youthful.

In a similar way, excessive sun exposure increases the risk of cataracts—a milky coating on the lens of the eye that can impair vision and ultimately lead to blindness. The role of the lens is to focus light onto the retina, the sensitive part of the eye that makes vision possible. So when the lens begins to turn opaque, it's like putting layers of whitewash on a window—it gets harder and harder to see through it.

Too much sun can also harm the immune system. There are special cells in the skin to detect invading organisms and trigger the immune response to them. But excessive ultraviolet (UV) rays in sunlight can damage this mechanism.

For all the same reasons, avoid tanning lamps and tanning salons, too.

Enjoy the Outdoors

Some may immediately protest: *What do you mean avoid the sun? Do I have to give up things I like, such as waterskiing and golf?* Of course not. We're not recommending that you hide out in a cave and emerge only during the dark hours. You can enjoy the sun and the outdoors all you want provided you do it safely, while protecting your skin.

Enjoy the Benefits of Sun Exposure

It's actually very important to get some sun exposure. Natural sunlight has many clear-cut and beneficial biological and psychological effects. For example:

- *Sunshine vitamin D.* In the normal diet, you consume chemicals that can be converted in your body into this essential vitamin. However, your body requires some sun exposure to accomplish this feat. Your body can't do it if you're indoors or in the dark all day.

- *Mood improvement.* As discussed in chapter 18, some people suffer from seasonal affective disorder (SAD), caused typically by too little sun exposure during the winter months when days are short, particularly at the more northern latitudes. One cure for SAD is a couple of hours or more per day of fresh, natural sunlight, which causes release in the brain of various hormones that make you feel happier.

- *Synchronizing biorhythms.* Regular sunlight exposure helps keep all your daily biorhythms in sync. If you ever experience jet lag, try getting bright sunlight exposure first thing in the morning in the new time zone (which may be the middle of the night, body time). The sunlight will rapidly trigger changes that help you adjust.

Protect Your Skin

We've said that too much sun is dangerous, yet we've touted the beneficial effects of natural light. How can you reconcile these seeming contradictions?

It's simple—go outside, enjoy outdoor activities, but protect your skin.

- *Use sunscreen.* There are two basic types: opaque barrier screens (sunblock) and chemical sunscreens (lotion). Though they work differently, both can be quite effective if strong enough. Strength is measured by the Skin Protection Factor (SPF), which refers to the number of minutes with the screen on that results in the same amount of damage as one minute with no screen. For example, an SPF of 10 means that you can wear it and stay in the sun for 10 minutes and yet get the effect of only 1 minute in the sun without protection. In other words, it's ten times safer than no protection. The experts recommend using sunscreens with SPF-15 or higher. SPF-15 means that it takes about 15 minutes with the sunscreen on to get the negative effect of only 1 minute if unprotected. You can play outside for a whole hour while protected and get the same risk as only four minutes if unprotected. So use high-SPF sunblock during all your lengthier outdoor activities under bright, direct sunlight. While you can find lotions with SPF-30 or even SPF-45, some experts believe they're no more valuable than SPF-15, though it certainly won't hurt you to use them.

- *Shade your skin.* The other approach is to enjoy your outdoor activities by sticking to the shade as much as possible. Ride your bike along the side of the street that's in the shade. Picnic under an open-walled pavilion with a roof. Bring your own "shade" by wearing a large straw hat or baseball cap that keeps the sun off your face. Do summer gardening or lawn mowing with a dark-colored, flimsy, but full-length shirt, gloves, and long pants. Add sunblock to the areas still uncovered—perhaps the neck and ears in this case. Experts used to recommend light clothing because it reflects the light and makes you feel cooler. But more recent work at the University of Nebraska Medical Center found that dark colors absorb more of the UV rays from sunlight, thus protecting the skin. You'll feel warmer, in other words, but be better protected. It's a good trade-off.

- *Check your skin.* As you undress, shower, and so on, periodically keep an eye on your skin. Look for the telltale signs, like changes in moles, that we discussed earlier. Have a spouse or significant other occasionally check the areas you can't see well, such as your back. If you catch a skin cancer and get it treated early enough, it's nothing to worry about.

Healthy skin not only looks good, but also provides a barrier that protects you from invasion by external disease organisms and dangerous chemicals in the environment. Protect your skin and it will protect you. For more information, consult the American Cancer Society's Web site: www.cancer.org.

CHAPTER 24

Watch Out for Environmental Hazards

W̶e would all like to live in a perfectly safe and healthy environment, but unfortunately that doesn't exist. Everywhere there are potential hazards. If you avoid one situation to eliminate one type of hazard, you'll end up in another location beset with its own risks. If you avoid all sun exposure through fear of solar radiation, you then stay indoors all the time and increase the risk of radon radiation.

You can't eliminate all risks and hazards, but you can minimize them, thus enhancing both the quality of your life and perhaps its duration.

Avoid Common Hazards in the Home

The Key to Home Safety

We could write an entire book just on specific home hazards and risks to health. Instead, let's summarize a sensible approach to assessing and correcting all major home risks in general. The key is to look around at what could go wrong and fix it before it does.

For instance, why leave that heavy canister of sugar close to the counter edge where someone could bump it off by accident, perhaps crushing a toe? If you note the carpet coming loose on one corner and bunching up, why leave it that way where someone may trip and fall? If there's only one tiny obstacle—say, a loose toy— anywhere in the house, you can bet that sooner or later someone will come along and stumble over it.

Toxins That Should Terrify

- *Food poisoning.* We mentioned food safety briefly in connection with spices in chapter 14. Now let's discuss it as an environmental risk. At least seventy-six million people a year get stomach cramps and diarrhea, or occasionally worse diseases, from tainted food. Salmonella poisoning alone catches about two million people a year. The most common cause is allowing a processed food, such as ham salad or egg salad, to sit at room temperature for many hours. Bacteria are everywhere in the environment, including on food handlers and preparers and in food. If food is stored hot (say, over canned heat at a buffet line) or cold (in the fridge or on ice), the bacteria don't proliferate to a dangerous level. But at room temperature—or outdoor picnic temperature—they multiply like crazy. It's best to prepare food just before you need it, or to store it in the fridge or freezer if there will be a long delay before consumption. Also, rinse fresh fruits, vegetables, and raw meat such as chicken before using them. Avoid cross-contamination caused by using the same dishes and utensils for clean and not-yet-cleaned food.

  Other food risks include the possibility of parasites in raw or improperly cooked food, like shellfish or pork, or seafoods taken from waters contaminated with chemical toxins or waste. Always buy food from known, reliable sources.

- *Allergens.* Ever suddenly get an unexplained itch or rash, swelling, burning or watery eyes, difficulty breathing, dizziness, any or all of the above? You may have an allergy. Perhaps you're aware of what you're allergic to. If so, great. You're ahead of the game and can actively seek to avoid it.

But perhaps you aren't sure about what you're allergic to. It could be dog or cat dander, dust mites in the home, the kind of detergent used in washing your clothes, or any of a thousand other possibilities. Keep experimenting (see page 122) until you track down the culprit and get rid of or minimize it. Some people think of allergies as trivial and don't worry about them. Sometimes, however, they can lead to more serious ailments. For instance, if an allergy causes sinus congestion, this can provide an ideal environment for bacteria or viruses to grow into a sinus infection or other more unpleasant disease.

- *Fungi.* The average home has a lot of molds, mildew, or other fungi. Some may be clearly visible, like the dark colony growing on your shower curtain or next to the kitchen sink. Some may be less visible—for instance, growing within your air ventilation system. Maybe it's time to vacuum out the vents and wipe them clean with a disinfectant. Replace the filter. Vacuum all your carpets frequently, too. You can eliminate a lot of allergens and many causes of disease with such simple steps.

Minimize Workplace Hazards

Sick-Building Syndrome

The name sounds a bit silly at first. After all, if a building is inanimate, how can it become ill? What this really means is that living creatures spending considerable time in the building frequently become ill. Both older and modern buildings often produce lots of allergies and illness. For instance, older ones may be more likely to harbor molds and mildew. Newer ones may be more likely to contain freshly made, painted, or coated furniture and other equipment that is off-gassing chemicals known to be allergenic. So when at home, clean, rearrange, and eliminate all you can of what bothers you.

Indoor Air Pollution

Most people don't realize that air pollution indoors is generally worse than outdoors. In some studies, the pollution exposure indoors is between five and seventy times worse than that outdoors. We bring all sorts of pollutants inside our buildings, often unwittingly, and they can't readily escape. For instance, hanging pest strips continually release pesticides into the air. If that occurs in a relatively small and confined space, then you'll be constantly breathing that stuff in. In some buildings, very little outside air gets in—there's a lot of weatherstripping to save on heating and cooling costs, and the air ventilation system may recycle mostly stale (or chemical-filled) air.

Another example is tobacco smoke. Even if your building has a separate designated area for smokers or even if they must smoke outside, it's possible for a considerable amount of smoke to reach the general ventilation system for everyone else. Similarly, attached or underground garages may funnel an incredible amount of automotive engine exhaust (including deadly carbon monoxide) into your building. Improperly vented space heaters also produce carbon monoxide. If fact, many people die from such exposures each year.

Some people think that air fresheners solve such problems. They don't. The various products sold as air fresheners basically just perfume the air, masking the odors of smoke or other fumes, but not eliminating any of them. In fact, masking may increase the risk by making us unaware of how bad the air we're breathing really is. Living green plants help a bit to improve air quality, mainly by turning carbon dioxide back into oxygen. But they can't remove all airborne pollutants.

Safety-Proof Your Life

Investigate

If you don't already know the environmental culprits that are bugging you, do a little research:

1. Make note of where you are and what you are doing every time you notice the same or similar symptoms. For instance, does it occur every time you mow the lawn or every time you sit in a certain position at your desk?

2. Experiment by changing one and only one element of your environment at a time. For example, try wearing a breathing mask when you mow the lawn, or moving your desk to a different position.

3. Note if this change makes a difference. If it does, then alter your environment or lifestyle accordingly. If it doesn't, scratch that hypothesis and try something else. You don't want to change two or more things at once, because then you may never know which one caused any possible variation in your response.

Keep Up-to-Date

The approach just described applies only to problems that show up right away. To avoid risky exposures that produce ill effects only years later, you must keep up with the latest scientific developments (through broadcast media and printed news) and apply common sense. For instance, if you microwave food in containers not meant for that purpose, you may release minor amounts of unpleasant chemicals from the plastic containers into the food. How do you know that future research won't prove those chemicals to be dangerous? Why risk it? You may not get sick right away, but doing a lot of this might increase your lifetime chances of contracting cancer somewhere down the line. Stick to using containers labeled *microwave safe* or *for microwave use*.

CHAPTER 25

Play the Detective and Catch 'Em Early

A lmost everybody likes detective stories and shows. It's thrilling to see the expert sift through the clues, track down leads, and eventually catch the bad guy just in the nick of time, before he or she can do further damage.

Similarly, you are the leading expert on your own body. You know better than anyone else what suddenly feels or looks different after all these years. And there are plenty of bad-guy diseases out there lurking in the shadows, ready to pounce. You should play the detective, note clues, follow up hunches, sniff out the trail, flush the bad guys out into the open, and zap them before they can do further harm. You will delay your biological clock and may save your life.

Examine Yourself to Catch Problems Early

A book of this length can't possibly provide an exhaustive list of all the possible health problems you should keep an eye out for. But we can discuss some of the most serious diseases and their most common warning signs. Not every occurrence of these signs necessarily indicates a major problem, however. Always consult your physician in cases of doubt.

General Signs Requiring Investigation

- *Sudden appearance.* Symptoms of more serious problems often appear rather suddenly—or at least are brought to your attention rather suddenly due to a quick worsening after a slow buildup.

- *Severity.* A symptom may be something you have experienced before (such as nausea, vomiting, or abdominal pain), but there's something unusually severe about this occurrence. It doesn't just seem to be a virus or stress this time, but something worse.

- *Long duration of the sign.* Pain or other symptoms from a slight injury or related problem will usually start to get better in three to five days if you take care of it properly. Something that seems to last and last or to get worse over time suggests a deeper, more serious problem.

- *That nagging suspicion.* Sometimes you (or your spouse or other loved one) will note your symptom and quickly suspect what it could be. You may be wrong, but it's usually worth checking it out.

Types of Diseases and Some Typical Signs

- *Heart disease.* Heart attacks kill hundreds of thousands of Americans every year. Classic warning signs include discomfort, tightness, or pain in the chest; numbness or pain in the arm; difficulty breathing; rapid or irregular heartbeat; or strong sweating, nausea, and dizziness. You don't have to experience all these signs, but there will usually be at least two or three. For instance, simple pain in the chest in the absence of any other symptom may merely reflect muscle soreness or cramping, perhaps in the pectoral (chest) muscles.

- *Stroke.* Early signals are sudden numbness, weakness, or paralysis in some body part, usually just on one side (e.g., the left arm or right foot only). There may also be mental confusion or loss of some behavioral skill such as vision or the ability to talk or read.

- *Diabetes.* There are different types of diabetes, including one that strikes suddenly in young children. But among people middle aged and older, with no prior history of diabetes, it usually strikes more slowly. It generally reveals itself in weight gain; more thirst, drinking, and urination than earlier in life; delayed healing time for even little things like skin cuts; and sexual impotence. A simple dipstick test can verify the presence of abnormally high levels of blood sugar (glucose) in the urine. A glucose tolerance test can verify whether the disease is present. Middle-aged people with a family history of diabetes should get screened regularly.

Cancer

Cancer is a special case: There are many kinds, and each has its own signs, usually in the body part with the cancer.

- *Colorectal cancer.* Signs include long-term bowel habit changes not related to diet changes, or long-term pain in the area. Blood in the stool is a common giveaway (although this can be caused in the short term by eating something like popcorn that has sharp edges). The blood may not be visible, however, so doctors recommend taking a fecal occult blood test every year once you hit middle age. This involves simply smearing a bit of stool on a test card for lab analysis. If you have any of the symptoms above and/or a family history of cancer in this region, your physician can check more thoroughly with a sigmoidoscopy, colonoscopy, or barium enema.

- *Bladder cancer.* Blood in the urine, particularly if accompanied by pain during urination, is the most common early sign. A reddish tinge to urine, however, is not always caused by blood. Eating a lot of red beets, for instance, can redden the urine, but this effect will certainly be temporary and not accompanied by pain. A persistent reddening and/or pain while urinating always merit a visit to your doctor.

- *Skin cancer.* This usually shows up as an unusual change in a mole or other peculiar growth on the skin. Please consult chapter 23 on the skin for more details.

- *Gender-related cancers.* For women, breast, uterine, and ovarian cancers are of special importance. Doctors recommend that all adult women check their breasts for lumps frequently throughout the year. Consult your physician if you find any unusual hard, knotty lumps. But don't panic if you find one—most are benign (harmless). Signs of other female cancers include abdominal pain that is otherwise unexplained and unusual menstrual-related bleeding.

  For men, prostate and testicular cancer are of particular concern. As men age, nearly all experience prostate enlargement, but this is often not cancerous. Among men who live long enough (eighty on up), however, the majority will experience prostate cancer eventually. On the other hand, many of these men never realize it, because it develops so slowly and has no serious symptoms among them. They die of other causes long before prostate cancer does them any real harm. This isn't to suggest that prostate cancer poses no hazards, of course. Among younger men, the disease is rarer but can be life threatening. Blood in the urine or pain in the genitals is often the first clue for either prostate or testicular cancer. Additional signs of the latter are a sudden change in the size (larger or smaller) of just one testicle, or the appearance of a lump or new growth on the testicle.

Knowing When to Consult Your Physician

You can play the detective, but don't try to be your own doctor, too. If you experience some of the warning signs discussed here or elsewhere from reliable sources and you feel worried, by all means consult your physician.

Even in the absence of warning signs, doctors recommend periodic checkups to catch any possible problems early. Some in the early stages won't show up in subjective symptoms but may reveal themselves in routine blood tests or other lab work or personal examination.

Recommendations for General Checkups

- If you're in your forties, every two to three years.

- When in your fifties, every two years.

- In your sixties or older, every year.

Recommendations for Specific Exams

Even without problem symptoms, these exams are recommended for those age fifty on up:

- *Eye exams, including glaucoma exam and retina check.* Every two to four years before age sixty-five, then every one to two years after that.

- *Blood pressure.* During every routine checkup, but at least once every year.

- *Blood tests, including blood cholesterol.* Every five years at least, assuming previous scores were healthy. If you score borderline or high at any time, then every year after that.

- *Colon exam.* Every three to five years.

- *Bone scan* (for those at risk for osteoporosis, particularly postmenopausal women not taking estrogen replacements). Get a Sahara test (which uses sound waves to measure the bone density in the heel) every three to five years.

- *Female exams.* Mammogram every year, and pap smear every one to three years.

- *Male exams.* Middle-aged men with a family history of prostate cancer, and all African American men even without symptoms or history, should get a PSA (prostate-specific antigen) test every year. (For unknown reasons, African American men have the highest rate of prostate cancer in the world.) Other middle-aged and older men should be screened once every two years.

For more information on general medical issues, symptoms of disease, and so forth, consult the following Web sites:

- http://www.intellihealth.com (a joint project by Johns Hopkins University Hospital and Aetna U.S. Healthcare).

- http://www.drkoop.com (named for the former U.S. surgeon general Dr. C Everett Koop).

- http://www.mayohealth.org (run by the Mayo Clinic).

CHAPTER 26

Immunize for Life

There are a lot of scary infectious diseases out there, such as hepatitis and pneumonia. True, the average life span has been increasing throughout this century, largely because medical science has conquered more and more contagious diseases. But a lot of them remain, and many of the older ones are resurging in newer and more virulent strains that are less responsive to our medical arsenal. The problem is that bacteria keep evolving into forms resistant to our antibiotics. Scientists keep developing new types of these wonder drugs, but bacteria continue to evolve in an endless race for supremacy. Some disease strains have developed resistance already to all but the newest and most powerful antibiotics.

Given that treatment of bacterial diseases is getting more difficult, and that antibiotics don't work on viral illnesses to begin with, doesn't it make sense to emphasize prevention rather than cure? It helps to practice normal sanitary habits such as avoiding contaminated food and water; washing your hands before eating, touching your eyes, or sticking fingers inside your nose, mouth, or ears; and minimizing contact with sick people (or at least washing up afterward). But since it's impossible to avoid all germs, the best prevention is immunization.

Immunization works by exposing your system to a little bit of a weakened or even killed pathogen such as bacteria or viruses. Your body then develops an immune response to the specific type of organism. If you encounter it later in ordinary life and the immune response is still strong, you can usually stop the organisms dead in their tracks, before they can launch a full-scale invasion. Think of your immune system cells as police officers or soldiers who literally identify, attack and destroy the bad guys.

For some immunizations such as tetanus, you must get periodic boosters or your immunity will gradually wear off. We recommend keeping an updated shot record in a secure place and following these guidelines for keeping each specific type of immunization up to date. It would really be a shame if you got your shots as a youth, failed to keep them up-to-date, and then got seriously ill as an adult due to this oversight.

Consider These Types of Immunizations

Some immunizations need only to be taken when you have already suffered a specific exposure. For instance, you need rabies vaccine only after you have been bitten by an animal that may be infected. Others should be taken in advance because of the widespread possibility of exposure or because the disease can progress too rapidly for immunization after exposure to protect you. Always consult your physician when deciding which vaccines to get.

The Old Standards

- *Flu.* Every winter, influenza sweeps the world and causes many deaths. In modern nations, millions get sick but few die, due to advanced treatment. Nevertheless, even here people who are older, weaker, or have compromised immune systems sometimes succumb. Your best bet to avoid the suffering and lost work time due to a nasty flu is to get a flu shot every year. Having one last year or five years ago may not help you much this year. The problem is that there are many, many variations on the flu. Any given shot usually protects you only from the three or so strains that public health authorities expect will be most common or serious in a particular year. Over time, if you take the shot each year, you may develop protection against twenty or thirty major strains. But if a new one emerges and you don't take the shot the year it's included, you could still catch it. So take your flu shot every year.

- *Tetanus.* You almost certainly received this several times while you were growing up. Please continue throughout life to get a booster about every ten years. Tetanus germs are all over the place, not just on dirty and rusty nails as we used to be taught. Any kind of puncture wound that goes fairly deep could put you at risk for tetanus. If you sustain such an injury and haven't had a vaccination in recent years, be sure to tell your doctor and get one. Despite the ready availability of tetanus shots, many Americans still contract the disease each year. And it's a terrible disease to get, with increasing paralysis and sometimes death. A single shot of a combined vaccine now can protect you from diphtheria as well as tetanus.

- *Polio.* An oral version of polio vaccine has been available for decades and is more pleasant to take than a shot. Nevertheless, many experts recommend the injectable vaccine instead, because it's more effective and carries no risk of transmitting polio rather than preventing it.

Newer, Emerging Immunizations

- *Hepatitis.* There are many forms of hepatitis, some contracted primarily through sexual contact or intravenous needles. For these forms, only people at risk, including medical personnel and drug users, and those traveling to countries with high rates of the disease, need the vaccinations. But other forms are found more widely in the population. For these, especially hepatitis B, everyone should get immunized unless they have specific immune system problems that put them at risk to the vaccine itself. Discuss this issue with your doctor if you have any questions. Certainly hepatitis—or liver infection— is one disease you want to avoid if at all possible. It can be very uncomfortable, recovery is slow, and there is sometimes permanent damage that necessitates dietary restrictions or other changes to your lifestyle.

- *Pneumonia.* This lung disease is less common and serious than it was fifty and a hundred years ago, but it still kills people every year. The lungs fill with fluid, and it becomes difficult to breathe. At best, a case of it will knock you flat on your rear for several days. Why risk all this when you can prevent it? Everyone over sixty-five, along with at-risk younger people (such as those with chronic health problems), should take the pneumococcal vaccine. Protection from a single shot lasts about five to ten years.

- *Chicken pox, measles, mumps.* Yes, we know these are childhood diseases. If you got them then, you're probably immune. But if you didn't, you can still contract these as an adult, when the symptoms are more severe. About a quarter million American adults get chicken pox every year. But there's no need to continue risking these diseases year after year: vaccinations are now available.

Nobody likes the pain of a shot. But that fleeting little pain is nothing compared to the suffering you can get from the disease it protects you from. Get your immunizations.

PART IV

Build Better Habits

In many ways, your personal habits are the prime determinants of how fast you age. You could inherit a very healthy body from your genes and early upbringing, yet waste it completely through bad habits as a young adult. Conversely, at this point you might have only average health, yet by developing a number of positive behavioral traits you could enhance health, reduce many of the biomarkers of aging, and greatly extend your life span.

In this section, we will deal first with the process of breaking entrenched bad habits, then with the kinds of bad habits you should break if you have them. Finally, we'll cover a number of good habits you should build or improve upon to further bust those various signs of age.

CHAPTER 27

Break Bad Habits

In part II (chapters 5 through 9), we spoke of changing unhealthy dietary practices, but how about all your other bad habits? Everyone has them! Whether it's smoking, drinking too much, taking foolish risks, nail biting, complaining excessively, overindulging in soap operas, yielding to temper outbursts, or playing practical jokes, we all do things we wish we didn't. In fact, we do them again and again, no matter how many times we regret it.

Consequences of Bad Habits

Even minor bad habits have a number of unpleasant effects:

- *They alienate others.* If it surprises you that relatives and companions find your hair chewing or off-color humor offensive, think of the many times that others' behavioral idiosyncrasies have perturbed you. You may think your little quirk is inoffensive, but theirs is really annoying. Please realize that their reaction is exactly the opposite. Your "little" peculiarity may be big to them!

- *You risk increased conflict and rejection.* When you rub others the wrong way repeatedly, the friction can produce heat.

You may trigger criticism, arguments, or rejection. Sometimes married couples are brought to the point of counseling and even divorce with most of their complaints involving behavioral traits that to the outside listener may seem minor and harmless. Ah, but to the people living with them day after day, such actions are crazy-making.

- *They stunt our maturity.* Every time we indulge a negative impulse we shouldn't, we reflect how immature we are. No one is perfect, of course, but growing maturity reflects itself in increased mastery over our impulses. If you see no sign of growth or, worse yet, see regression in your own behavior, then you're doing something wrong.

- *Some bad habits accelerate our biological clocks.* While some habits are, in fact, relatively harmless, others have repercussions for our physical and/or mental health. Repeatedly eating too much fat and total calories increases obesity and the risk of some pretty dreadful diseases. Conversely, gaining control over habits such as these can improve your health and lengthen your life span.

Changing Bad Habits

We're not going to pretend that changing habits is always easy. But it can be done. In fact, you almost certainly have done it before, even if you don't remember exactly when or how. For instance, as a teenager, were you a bit nervous around members of the opposite sex, perhaps hemming and hawing on the phone while trying to get a date? The embarrassment after several experiences of this probably made you determined to act more polished in the future, so you practiced silently, or aloud in private, or with a friend until you could get your comments out minus all the stammering. If you could change your behavior then, you can do it again now.

Psychiatrists and psychologists have formalized into therapy a number of techniques based ultimately on applied common sense and personal experience. The professionals practice these, certainly, in a more consciously systematic and organized way. But parents, among others, have also used some of these same approaches since time immemorial. We've even popularized some of these methods with little folk sayings to help us remember them. For example, "If you fall off a bike, get right back on again." Your mother probably told you something like that when you were ten or twelve. The point was that if you end an experience with a painful failure, you'll have trouble trying the sport or activity again. Rather than let fear wrap its paralyzing tentacles around you, you need to leave yourself with a taste of victory, with a self-label as a winner in your heart. Mental health professionals have taken this simple notion and researched every nuance out of it and developed systematic techniques to help you solve far more serious problems.

First Steps

- *Realize you have a problem.* If you remain unaware of a bad habit, you're unlikely to change it. Practice a little insight. If you experience a certain unpleasant reaction in social relationships again and again, think back to what you were doing that might have triggered it. If you still can't figure it out, consider asking the other person, "Did I do something to offend you? I didn't mean to. What was it?"

- *Get motivated.* In most cases, you won't need to ask. Most people are fully aware of their bad habits. Their problem instead is the inability to control them. Build a case in your own mind for making the change and remind yourself of it frequently. For instance, "Marge hates it when I leave the toilet seat up. I love Marge. I must remember next time to lower it again." Nothing facilitates behavior better than strong motivation.

- *Develop a plan.* Figure out why you repeat a certain misbehavior. Where's the reward, the payoff? Try to get that reward in some other way. Turn to one of the bad-habit busters below to rid yourself of the negative conduct once and for all. You may not achieve instantaneous or complete relief, but you should experience some improvement. Even if you slip back one step for every two forward, don't grow too discouraged as long as your net progress continues in the right direction.

- *Get help if necessary.* If you try everything else suggested here and still find no relief at all, get help. Depending on the problem, consult a trusted friend or family member, or perhaps seek professional help, as from a cleric, therapist, or other counselor. Don't be ashamed to get help if you need it.

Habit Busters

No one technique works all the time for everyone with every type of problem. Depending upon the habit you want to change, you might use one approach for fear of insects and a very different approach for losing your temper.

- *Desensitization.* For habits involving anxieties and fears— say, of public speaking, flying, or handling major equipment at work—try this one. First, make a list of all the major aspects of the situation that disturb you. Next, rank these aspects from the least threatening to the scariest. Then, employ the relaxation techniques discussed in chapters 4 and 50 to stay relaxed while thinking about the mildest aspect. Repeat this over time until you can stay relaxed while thinking about it. Days or weeks later (however long it takes), repeat the process with the next scariest aspect. Over time, work your way all the way up the scale.

- *Time-outs.* For habits involving giving in to sudden impulses, such as anger or the desire to nosh down a second piece of pie, try this. If possible, just freeze in place for a moment and force yourself to think about what you're about to do. In the case of snacking, remind yourself of that famous saying, "A moment on the lips; a lifetime on the hips." Still want it? Promise yourself you can have it in thirty minutes if you still feel hungry then. In most cases, by that time your stomach will have processed the first piece of pie enough to tell your brain that you're already full.

- *Replacement therapy.* This is usually quicker than desensitization and can be used to strengthen the power of time-outs. But it can only be tried if you can come up with a suitable alternative. What you need is a better behavior that conflicts with or displaces the action you want to change. For example, some people find that chewing gum helps prevent the desire to smoke or overeat. Drinking a lot of water or taking a walk reduces the urge to snack.

As you attempt to change your bad habits, try to be patient with others who are trying to change their own.

CHAPTER 28

Give Up Tobacco

Tobacco use kills about twelve hundred Americans a day (about half a million a year)—more than all the U.S. combat deaths in World War II and Vietnam combined, more than all the deaths on the nation's highways. Smoking disfigures people, robs them of the ability to breathe, racks their bodies with agonizing diseases, and cuts years or even decades off their lives. It makes them smelly, it discolors teeth, it impairs their enjoyment of food. Research recently published in the *Journal of the American Medical Association* reports previously unknown risks even to hearing, with smokers 70 percent more likely to experience hearing loss than nonsmokers. If you think smoking is cool, sophisticated, and debonair, go visit a longtime smoker in the hospital who's dying of lung cancer that has metastasized to the brain. Your opinion will change very quickly.

How Smoking Slashes Years Off Your Life

All Tobacco Is Dangerous

Some people think that only cigarettes are harmful. They say, "I smoke cigars or a pipe; I don't inhale; therefore, my smoking is

safe." Others say, "I don't smoke at all. I just gnaw on chewing tobacco or keep a wad of snuff between my gums and cheek; since
there's no smoke, it's safe."

Sorry, but none of these myths is true. Inhaling smoke may be
worse for the lungs, but bringing tobacco's poisons into your mouth
in any form creates terrible risks. Just as the toxins and carcinogens
in smoke attack lung tissue, the same tobacco ingredients in the
mouth attack all parts of the oral cavity and surrounding tissues.
The individual cell under attack doesn't care if the harmful chemicals came as smoke or as dissolved in saliva. Poison is poison. And
cancer of the jaw or throat is just as scary as lung cancer.

Tobacco Increases Health Risks

Someone else will say, "Not true! My uncle smoked all his life
and lived until the age of ninety-three."

It's correct that not everyone who uses tobacco dies from it, but
the risks are very large and very real. If six people play Russian
roulette by placing one bullet in a revolver with six chambers, then
each in turn points at his or her head and pulls the trigger, not
everyone suffers, but one is going to die. Habitual tobacco users
really are taking a risk just as obvious and dangerous in the long
term as this.

What makes you think you're the smoker who'll live to ninety-
three? What if you're the one who loses twenty years of life instead?

Smoking not only cuts short the average smoker's life, but also
significantly impairs his or her enjoyment even while alive. Smoke
doesn't simply affect the obvious organs such as mouth and lungs.
The nicotine, tar, and other toxic substances get into the bloodstream, where they can attack all your organs. They increase the
risk of heart attacks and strokes. Smoking can even interfere with
sexual function and fertility.

If there's no real reward or payoff for taking the risk, why
take it?

Tobacco Is Habit Forming

Smoking quickly can become a habit—it feels uncomfortable to quit. At this point, you're addicted, and trying to forsake the weed lends to withdrawal symptoms and cravings. There are ways around this problem, however (see below).

The Benefits of Quitting

The good news is that if you stop smoking, your health will in most cases begin to improve almost immediately. If you quit early enough, you may be able to recover almost all of your lung capacity and presmoking health. The exception to this good news occurs when you've already developed a potentially fatal disease before you quit, though even then quitting improves your odds of successful therapy and survival.

Quitting lessens the impact of secondhand smoke on your loved ones as well. Nonsmokers who live with heavy smokers face greatly increased risks to their own health. For example, heart attacks are four times more common among nonsmokers living with heavy smokers than among those living with other nonsmokers.

Don't Wait—Quit Now!

How to Quit Comfortably

If you can quit cold turkey, do it. But most people can't. As Mark Twain used to say, "It's easy to quit smoking; I've done it hundred of times."

- *Ease withdrawal.* Put on the patch, chew the gum, try the filters that cut down on nicotine intake—it is okay to try the products designed to help people quit. Gradually reducing intake lessens the withdrawal discomfort. But it does spread this discomfort out over a longer period.

- *Avoid activities associated with smoking.* If to you the weekly poker game, happy hour at Joe's Bar, or Saturday-night boxing is associated with smoking, then avoid these activities—at least until you feel secure about quitting.

- *Don't let smoking friends draw you back in.* Smokers sometimes hate to see someone else quit and will try to bring you back into the fold by offering free tobacco. Say no politely but firmly. If they won't accept you as a nonsmoker, maybe it's time for some new friends.

- *Replace the old habits with new ones.* If you spent years not only smoking but also thinking about tobacco, purchasing tobacco, handling tobacco, and so on, you need some new activities to replace these old habits. It can be as simple as chewing sugarless gum, knitting, or, better yet, exercising more.

- *If you give in, don't give up.* Okay, so you slip up now and then. No one is perfect. Don't beat yourself up about it. Just try again to quit. Even a partial or incomplete quitting is a step in the right direction. Take another step.

Avoid the Weight Gain Associated With Quitting

People who quit smoking often gain weight, sometimes so much that they take up the habit again. Not a good plan. Both conditions are hazardous to your health, so don't trade either one for the other.

Experts differ on why quitting causes weight gain. Do ex-smokers just eat more because they're nervous? Do they eat more because the food tastes better without their taste buds clogged with tar and smoke? Do their metabolisms slow down without all the nicotine revving them up? Maybe a combination of all of the above?

Whatever the ultimate answers to those questions, you can avoid undue weight gain when you quit by following the advice given in other chapters of this book:

- Exercise more (chapter 2).

- Eat a balanced diet (chapter 5).

- Consume less fat (chapter 6).

- Replace junk food with healthier snacks (chapters 7, 9, 17, and more).

One of the most important things you can do to slow your biological clock, to lengthen your life span, and to add enjoyment to your years is to quit tobacco.

CHAPTER 29

Prevent Pink Elephants

You can read on one page of the newspaper about the health benefits of alcohol, and on another about its deadly health hazards; there probably is no other subject on which modern research is so confusing.

This isn't the fault of the researchers, because people on both sides of the issue are probably correct. Beverage alcohol can have a wide range of effects, depending upon how it's used. One person's use may enhance health, while another person's may lead to death. Let's examine both sides of this controversy.

The Health Benefits of Alcohol

Taken in moderation (as defined below), alcohol has some potential benefits:

- *Alcohol can protect the circulatory system.* It can reduce the risk of heart disease, heart attacks, and strokes. Long-term moderate users have far fewer heart attacks than teetotalers (or alcoholics, for that matter). Some research suggests that wine is better at this than either beer or hard liquor, and that red wine is better than white. But other research suggests that alcohol itself, regardless of the beverage type that contains it, is helpful. For instance, a study at the University of Wisconsin–Madison Medical School of nearly a thousand older diabetics found that moderate alcohol consumption regardless of source (whiskey, wine, or beer) reduced the risk of coronary heart disease by up to 80 percent. Another study at the Columbia University College of Physicians and Surgeons in New York found a 45 percent lower risk of ischemic stroke (the kind caused by blockage rather than rupture of a blood vessel in the brain) among light drinkers, regardless of beverage type.

It may be that both contentions are true, that alcohol does help, and that the additional ingredients in red wine help even more. The latest research at Cornell University and the University of California, Davis, suggests that the chemical in red wine that's most helpful is resveratrol. Plain red grapes and grape juice, however, as well as other foods, can provide some of this and the related flavonoid compounds without undergoing fermentation to alcohol.

- *Alcohol facilitates digestion.* This is particularly true of wine drunk with a meal.

- *Other benefits.* Some research suggests that wine may even help reduce the risk of such disparate diseases as cancer and kidney stones.

The Health Hazards of Alcohol

Given what we've just said, are you thinking it's time to stock your home bar up to the ceiling? On the contrary, excess alcohol poses great dangers that far outweigh the helpful effects of moderate use. Thus most experts, even when fully aware of the benefits, never go so far as to actually recommend that nondrinkers take up alcohol. They know there's always a certain proportion of new drinkers who will develop full-blown alcoholism and die of it. Excessive alcohol is one of our major killers today. Here's some examples:

- *Increased accidents.* Perhaps best known are the lethal effects of drunk driving, still one of the major causes of highway deaths despite widespread campaigns against it. Less well known is that all categories of accidental injuries and deaths—from drownings to falls—are increased by inebriation.

- *Cirrhosis of the liver.* Since this vital organ is the one that detoxifies the body of alcohol, heavy drinking wears it out. In long-term alcoholics, it often fails, killing them.

- *Other diseases.* Heart disease, cancer, and more are all increased by alcohol abuse.

- *Relationship problems.* Problem drinkers typically have serious difficulties at work and with family and friends. Spousal and child abuse are all too common when someone is inebriated.

- *Mental illness.* Excess alcohol attacks the brain and can render the long-term abuser psychotic, with a dysfunctional memory and loss of ability to handle ordinary life. Such alcoholics begin to have hallucinations—seeing, hearing, or feeling things that aren't really there, including the proverbial "pink elephants."

How Much Is Safe?

This is the key question. A little bit may be actually good for you. A little bit more is *not* better for you. A lot more is very bad for you. So where do you draw the line?

When you drink, alcohol enters the bloodstream and spreads through all the organs and tissues. Therefore, the larger you are, the more body mass you have, the less the effect of a drink on any single organ, like your brain. In general, men tend to be larger and can safely accommodate up to two or three drinks per day. Women usually tend to be lighter, and only about one or two drinks per day is recommended as a maximum. But even when sticking to these safety limits, drinking every day can build a habit that for some will lead to alcoholism later.

Defeating Alcohol Dependency

Recognizing Dependency

The first step toward solving a drinking problem is to become aware that you have it. You must admit to yourself that you've lost control. Here are some signs of having some type of alcohol dependency, from its milder forms of habitual overdrinking all the way up to full-blown (and commonly lethal) alcoholism:

- *Needing to drink every day.* Feeling nervous and anxious if unable to get a drink; highly upset if no alcohol is available.

- *Drinking alone.* We don't mean by this someone who occasionally has a drink while dining alone, but rather those who prefer to be alone so that they can drink all they want without being observed.

- *Frequently drinking with the intention of getting high or drunk.* Social drinkers may occasionally get carried away in the spirit of a party and have one or two more than they should. But the hard drinker deliberately downs as much as possible as fast as possible in the conscious attempt to get inebriated.

- *Frequently overdrinking with the goal of forgetting problems and worries.*

- *Loss of control over the amount drunk.* The person may intend to stick to two or three drinks, but once this limit is reached has no control and just keeps slugging away until totally inebriated.

- *Blackouts, passing out, memory lapses.* Those who wake up from a drinking binge and don't know how they got where they are or what they did the night before had way, way too much to drink.

Get Help

If you have a problem with alcohol abuse and realize it, get help. Join Alcoholics Anonymous or similar group; see a pastor, priest, or rabbi who has been trained in the counseling of alcoholics; go to a clinic or medical professional; find a relative or close friend who will join you in the fight. Maybe you'll need to try all the above. But do something, and the sooner the better. Tobacco and excess alcohol habits are two key ways to accelerate your biological clock, making you look years older and cutting years off your life. Beat these two dependencies, if you have either or both, before they defeat you!

CHAPTER 30

Unplug the TV

Notice we didn't say, "Toss the TV in the trash." TV does have its merits. After a really hard day at work or slaving in the home, who hasn't enjoyed occasionally kicking back with the remote and vegging out in that soft glow? And who among us doesn't appreciate the ease with which TV connects us to the outside world, with news, weather reports, and special cultural events brought right into our living rooms?

But like so many things, it's easy to overdo TV. Just as some people eat too much or drink too much, some watch too much TV (as defined and assessed by the questionnaire below). To people like this we say, turn off the set! Unplug it. Get outside and do something else—exercise, talk on the phone, meet friends, go out for dinner, volunteer in the community, write a poem, read.

Turning into a couch potato is not healthy. Research shows that people who watch a lot of TV tend to be obese—for several reasons. First, inactivity means you're expending fewer calories. Second, people tend to snack a lot more while watching the tube. Haven't you noticed that ads for snack foods are among the most common on TV? The problem is worse for growing youngsters. According to the Baylor College of Medicine, one-quarter of kids watch four or more hours of television each day; the more TV watched, the fatter the kids tend to be. Though worse for youth, this is also a problem for adults. The University of Minnesota's School of Public Health studied for a year more than a thousand people who were trying to control their weight. The more TV they watched that year, the more weight they gained.

Excessive viewing can also distort your perceptions of the outside world, making viewers more fearful about crime, more irritable, and more aggressive. Getting excited about a sporting event, for instance, can raise your blood pressure considerably without leading to the real exercise that would allow you to work off that aroused tension and excitement.

Excessive TV attachment can ruin family and other social life and generally mess up your value system. One survey conducted by the advertising agency D'Arcy Masius Benton & Bowles and reported in *TV Guide* found that when asked what their greatest pleasures in life were, people listed TV in first place. It was cited by 68 percent—more folks than listed friends, helping others, or vacationing. Another survey conducted for *TV Guide* by Peter D. Hart Research Associates, Inc., asked people if they would give up TV forever in exchange for large sums of money. Forty-six percent said they wouldn't do it for anything less than a million dollars, and a quarter wouldn't stop even for that.

Some of our slang reveals just how absorbing TV can be. For instance, we refer to a woman whose husband devotes himself to TV athletics as a "sports widow." Similarly, we often call the glowing box a "boob tube," for its well-known effects of robbing youngsters of the creativity and imagination that can be found in active play.

How to Tell If You Watch Too Much

Surveys show that many young people spend more time watching TV than attending school. Many adults spend more of their waking hours watching TV than doing anything else other than work. Instead, strike a happy balance between being a TV shunner and a TV addict. Where do you draw the line? Take this self-quiz.

Subjective Signs of Watching Too Much

- Is your most important reading of the week your TV program guide?

- Do you build your after-work schedule around your program timetable (as opposed to just turning the television on now and then when not much else is going on)?

- Are you willing to postpone almost any other activity in order to watch even a show that isn't that good?

- Do you spend a lot of time buying (or thinking about buying) all sorts of TV-related gizmos and enhancements—ever-larger TVs, satellite dishes, and cable packages with many dozen different channels? Do you find that the more of these things you get, the more you still want?

- Do you complain a lot about TV quality yet still watch just as much as always?

Interpersonal Signs of TV Excess

- Does your spouse or primary companion complain frequently that you watch too much TV?

- Do you abandon friends or refuse to make them so that you can spend more time watching television?

- When you're with friends and colleagues, is your main source of conversation the shows you recently watched or upcoming ones you want to watch?

Objective Measures of Excessive Watching

- Do you watch several hours of TV every day without fail?

- Are you ever late to work or to other appointments or very tired throughout the day because you watched TV late the night before and just couldn't turn it off?

- Do you frequently fall asleep with the TV on?

- Is the rest of the house a mess, but the TV corner spotless like a shrine?

Give yourself one point for each yes answer. If you scored more than one or two, please consult the next section on how to regain control.

Cut Down on TV Watching

If the previous self-quiz revealed that you're a TV addict, here are some suggestions for ways to reduce your dependence without going cold turkey.

- At least one night a week, leave the TV off altogether. If you need the news or weather report, get it from the radio or the newspaper. Unplug the TV if that helps you resist the temptation to just grab the remote and plop into an easy chair for the rest of the evening.

- Most days, limit yourself to two hours or less of TV.

- Reserve your watching time for shows in which you really have an interest. If there's nothing that good on, don't complain, just turn off the set. Instead, talk to someone, visit with friends, read, do a crossword puzzle, or practice a hobby.

- Make sure you find time for stretching and exercise, social and emotional life, intellectual stimulation, and adequate rest before turning on the tube.

In short, don't allow yourself to be a slave to TV. Become its master. This can add, in effect, several years to your active life. Don't believe it? Look at this example: Bill Smith used to watch thirty-five hours of TV a week, but now has cut down to fifteen.

He's saved twenty hours a week for more useful and more beneficial activities such as exercise and social relationships. Twenty
hours a week times just fifty weeks a year (we're rounding off for
simplicity) makes a thousand hours a year saved. Multiply that by,
say forty years, and Bill has saved forty thousand hours in the rest
of his adult life. There's only about six thousand waking hours in a
year, so Bill has added, in effect, nearly seven years of active life
(forty thousand total hours divided by six thousand hours). Think
of what *you* could accomplish with seven, five, or even two more
years of active life!

CHAPTER 31

Avoid Unnecessary Risks

How good are you at accurately perceiving risk? Choose the riskier alternative from each pair below:

1. Living next to (a) a nuclear power plant or (b) a coal-powered plant?

2. Traveling across country by (a) commercial plane or (b) private automobile?

3. Eating vegetables grown (a) using commercial pesticides or (b) organically at home?

Most people pick (a) in the items above, but the correct answer is (b). For example, in item 1 above, most people don't realize that with all the safety controls, U.S. nuclear power plants have never released harmful levels of radiation, not even in the so-called worst U.S. incident ever—the one at Three Mile Island in Pennsylvania in 1979. Burning coal not only creates noxious fumes but actually releases more radiation (which is a contaminant in coal) into the environment than the average nuclear power plant. Similarly, about forty thousand people die every year on the nation's highways, but far fewer die in U.S. commercial aircraft accidents (even counting the horrible terrorist attacks of September 11, 2001). The answer to the third question above is explained in the "Natural versus artificial" section below.

Why do we so often estimate risk inaccurately?

The Irony of Risk Perception

Reasons for Misperceiving Risks

- *The media exaggerate some risks while overlooking others.* The rare air crash makes big headlines, but the thousands of auto accidents rarely do (unless they involve a princess or someone else famous). In recent years, the media have terrified the entire nation about the danger of the fungicide alar on apples (which is negligible) or cyanide found in a couple of Chilean grapes only once, nearly destroying entire industries in the process. At the same time, the media consider the ordinary risks that claim life and limb daily (bathtub falls, stair trips, home fires) not to be very newsworthy at all.

- *People fear things they have no control over more than those they do.* As a mere passenger in an airplane, the typical person feels out of control and exaggerates fears of a possible accident. The same person behind an automobile wheel feels more in control and thus safer, even though he or she actually has no command over the many hazards on the road (such as drunk drivers, lumber falling off trucks, and careless speeders).

- *Choice in risk.* People tend to underestimate the risks for activities they voluntarily choose, like smoking cigarettes. They tend to overestimate the hazards in things forced on them, such as pesticides used on food by the big agricultural companies.

- *Natural versus artificial.* People think that artificial chemicals such as pesticides are far more dangerous than natural ones, even though chemically there may be no difference. Bruce Ames of the University of California at Berkeley estimates that we consume ten thousand times more natural pesticides than artificial ones—yet neither should be a source of concern.

The Consequences of Misperception

- *Misperceiving risks makes disasters more likely.* When people think they're safe, they take fewer precautions. Since all the possible traps are still there, such people are more likely to fall into one.

- *Avoiding a smaller risk may make a larger one more likely.* People who shun fruit due to exaggerated fears of pesticides may greatly increase heart disease risk from a poor diet.

- *Misjudging danger adds stress to your life.* One heinous crime in the news can make all of us feel less safe in our own neighborhoods, even though such a crime is unlikely to occur there. People who watch a lot of TV often harbor exaggerated fears of crime that limit their freedom, activities, and peace of mind.

Develop More Accurate Perceptions of Risk

The best way to accomplish this is to read, to stay informed. Read reliable newspapers, magazines, and journals rather than tabloids. Consult experts about things that trouble you. If you're vexed continually about a skin mole that has changed color, have your doctor check it out. Either you'll find your fear was correct and have your cancer treated, or you'll learn it's nothing and finally be relieved about it. Either way you win.

Reduce Risks

Some people actively seek out risk. They get an adrenaline high from doing something hazardous like speeding around sharp curves or diving off bridges into unknown waters. Sooner or later, gamblers like this are going to lose. They may forfeit everything. And no amount of adrenaline thrills will make up for losing a leg, a loved one, or a life.

If you need that adrenaline high, get it in the safest ways possible—like in organized sports or at a well-run amusement park. Avoid unnecessary risks altogether. This alone can prevent painful injuries or an impaired ability to enjoy life. It can also add years to your active and happy life span.

Here are some easy ways to avoid life-threatening risks:

- *Take medical tests.* Don't let fear of the test or what the test might reveal keep you from taking it. Yes, some tests are inconvenient or uncomfortable, but the alternative may be far worse if you fail to catch the illness that the test is designed for. For instance, some people are so scared of radiation that they refuse to accept X rays. Some are too embarrassed to go in for their pap smears.

- *Follow treatment guidelines.* For instance, if your doctor finds cancer and recommends radiation therapy or chemotherapy, by all means get a second opinion. But if the experts agree that such therapies are the best way to save your life, don't let fear of the treatments hold you back.

- *Don't follow the crowd.* Let's say everybody else in your group wants to try *fugu* (the blowfish sushi that can be fatally poisonous if not correctly prepared). If you don't genuinely want to try it, don't let them talk you into doing it. If you don't feel like skydiving with your friends, then don't, regardless of what they say about it.

- *Avoid recreational drugs.* They're simply too dangerous in every conceivable way.

- *Follow directions when using industrial chemicals.* Ditto for household cleansers, solvents, and other chemicals. Some of these are quite toxic. Before using, read carefully the instructions on the label and follow them. For instance, solvents should always be used in well-ventilated areas, because a buildup of fumes in an enclosed space can be quite dangerous.

- *Quit smoking.* The average smoker loses six years of life. See chapter 28 for help.

- *Lose excess weight.* People who are overweight by 15 percent lose on average two years of life. Greatly overweight people may lose decades. See chapter 5 for help.

- *Enjoy a happy marriage.* Married people live, on average, five years longer than single ones. Just make sure you marry someone compatible to minimize the risk of divorce. And see chapter 42 for ways to keep romance alive.

- *Avoid alcoholism.* Heavy drinkers lose at least one year of life on average. A true alcoholic may cut decades off his or her life. See chapter 29 for help.

- *Wear seat belts.* For drivers in auto accidents, those wearing seat belts have a 42 percent less chance of dying than those who don't.

- *Wear protective sports gear.* When bicycling or motorcycling, wear a helmet. If using in-line skates, wear your knee pads.

Many people who are aware of ideas like these still can't seem to follow them. But you shouldn't give in so easily. Take control of your life. Force yourself to do the sensible thing.

You'll be glad you did.

CHAPTER 32

Simplify Your Life

Some people's lives are so hectic that they've decided to just chuck it all. No more lengthy commute. No more noisy, crowded, hostile city. No more high-pressure seven-to-seven career. They cash in their stock options, sell off their deluxe condos, buy a spacious farm in the woods, and try to earn a living as a farmer, writer, or craftsperson.

This daydream appeals to so many because they have made their lives far too complex and stressful. But you don't have to completely abandon your current life to regain your sanity. You can begin to make your current life more manageable, thus reducing stress, enhancing enjoyment of life, and prolonging your youthful vigor.

Roles and Scripts

All of us play many roles in life—child, spouse, parent, employee, community leader. Each role bears certain responsibilities and requires the commitment of time and energy. We fulfill roles by accepting scripts that tell us how to play these roles. In most cases (other than certain jobs and professional positions), these scripts are informal and unwritten rather than officially codified. We acquire these scripts over the years often in a subconscious way, from observing and imitating others such as parents, teachers, and friends.

Sometimes we accept unrealistic scripts that are impossible to fulfill. For instance, some women strive simultaneously to be a full-time professional, a full-time wife, and a full-time mother (in short, "Super Mom"). They feel constantly exhausted from trying to do the work of three people. We aren't counseling you to neglect your proper responsibilities and commitments. But we do suggest that you reconsider how you fulfill them and think carefully before accepting new ones. Here are some ideas.

Twelve Ways to Simplify

1. Rewrite Your Scripts

Think rationally about your life. If you have developed an unrealistic and unnecessary script over the years, rethink it. Change it! If this activity isn't something formally agreed to, you don't necessarily have to do it. For instance, just because your mother baked fresh bread every day doesn't mean you have to. If you want to, great. But if it's a painful burden and you're sick of it, explain to your family the reason for the change and then make it.

2. Prioritize Your Fundamental Commitments

A religious person might list these, in order, as "God, family, job, community." Someone else might give lip service to "family first" yet live as a workaholic who clearly places job first. Different people hold different values. Think through your own and establish conscious priorities so that in any given conflict, you'll know what to decide.

3. Decline Excess Tasks

You did a superb job planning, organizing, and running the PTA Christmas party. The PTA president pats you on the back and invites you to start working on the summer picnic next. You don't know where you'll find that extra five or ten hours a week, but feeling on the spot and unwilling to offend, you grudgingly accept.

Wrong! Think before you automatically accept such offers. If you want to and have the time, fine. But if you don't, then politely decline. Suggest that it's someone else's turn next.

4. Drop Excess Organizations

You can't belong to and support every group in town. Prioritize them. Devote yourself to the ones you deem truly important. Drop the lower-priority ones when you can, being sure first to fulfill any lingering commitments already made. (It's not nice to add to someone else's stress by just skipping out.)

5. Don't Compete Unnecessarily

Forget about keeping up with the Joneses. Just because they have three cars doesn't mean you have to take on another part-time job so you can afford a third one also. Set your own goals and work toward them; don't let others write your goals for you.

6. Cut Out Avoidable Work

Obviously, a paying job is highly important. You must devote considerable time, talent, and energy to doing a good job so you can keep your position and hope to move higher. But are you doing more than you really need to, at the expense of other worthy priorities such as family or personal health? For some people, particularly those in families with two or more wage earners, perhaps working part time is the answer.

7. Delegate

Ask for the help of others. At work, spread tasks around to equalize workloads if you can. Train the children to help out around the home. Many parents say, "It's much too hard to get Jimmy or Suzy to make the bed or wash the dishes. It's easier to do it myself." That can become a self-fulfilling prophecy. If you invest the time to train and discipline your children when young (when, yes, it would be easier to do it yourself), this will pay dividends later in better performance as they mature.

8. Shed Useless Items

We acquire a lot of junk throughout our lives. Of course, when we first save something, we don't normally think of it as junk. If it remains important to us, we never come to think of it that way. But a lot of items do lose their personal value for us, yet we cling to them out of habit and spend a lot of unnecessary time and money caring for them. Instead, sell off or give away something you don't really want anymore, whether a collection of china or an unused boat or that little cabin in the woods that you don't even enjoy.

9. Move

Maybe you live in a much larger house than you need, especially if your kids have grown up and left. Why keep working to clean, heat, and pay a share of the mortgage on rooms you're not even using? This isn't for everyone, but for some, maybe a move to a smaller or more convenient house would help simplify your life.

10. Don't Burn the Candle at Both Ends

If you overdo for too long, you may burn yourself out. You may become incapable of maintaining even normal levels of performance. Strive to get adequate rest and relaxation (see chapter 36).

11. Face Reality

If it becomes clear that your self-expectations are unrealistic, don't keep beating your head against the wall trying to meet them; change your expectations in a more realistic direction. This isn't to deny the importance of high goals, but don't psychologically beat yourself up over every seeming failure to meet them. Not everyone can become an Academy Award–winning actor, an NBA All-Star, or a "Super Dad."

12. Don't Throw Out the Baby

Don't read the above eleven suggestions as meaning you should withdraw from life or start dying piece by piece by shutting down the corridors of your life. On the contrary, to slow your biological clock you must remain active, vibrant, and vivacious as long as you can. But if your life is too busy, just cut down to a manageable level.

All of the above probably sounds easier than it really is to put into practice. But remember that trying to simplify your life is not an all-or-nothing proposition. You'll benefit from taking even small steps in this direction, even if they're only temporary. Almost anything beats feeling overburdened and pressured constantly, all the time. See also the next three chapters for more ideas about how to gain some control over the stresses in your life.

CHAPTER 33

Manage Your Time

An important part of mastering your life is to gain better control of time. Even though we all have the exact same amount of time in each twenty-four-hour day, some of us waste a good portion of it and have a hard time getting anything done. Others are more adept at squeezing everything in.

Avoid These Ten Time Wasters

1. *"I'll do it later."* All of us tend to procrastinate, but some worse than others. Some people seem incapable of finishing any major task because they just keep putting it off. As the old saying goes, a journey of a thousand miles begins with the first step. Force yourself to take that first step and things will start to fall into place.

2. *Conveniently forgetting about something important.* Some people manage to let important things slip below their radar. When they don't get it done, they think the excuse "I forgot" will suffice. It's better to make sure you remember and then follow through. (More on memory enhancement in chapter 37.)

3. *Handling the same item more than once.* Some people like to spend a lot of time organizing everything they have to do that day. They'll look through all their tasks, think about them a lot, sequence them by priority, and then go take an extended coffee break without ever really starting anything. Scheduling and organizing are very good if they lead to productive work. But if tinkering with the schedule endlessly becomes a way to avoid work, then forget it. Dump the schedule and just plunge in and do something. Don't pore over something for an extended period and then lay it aside for later. If you're going to take more than a second or two deciding what to do with it, just go ahead and finish it off right then and there.

4. *Splintering concentration.* During hectic periods, it's easy to try to do too many things at once. You rush from the computer to the phone to the typewriter to a meeting to the phone to an interruption. . . . When people are descending upon you like a horde of locusts all at once, you can't help it. But if you're jumping back and forth among multiple competing tasks when you don't have to, don't. Grab hold of something and stick with it until you take care of it. Then go to something else. Splintering your focus makes mistakes more likely and allows you to forget something altogether.

5. *Dwelling on the unimportant.* Sometimes it's easier to avoid the really important big jobs by making ourselves feel busy on the simple or trivial ones. There's nothing wrong with getting your day started with a couple of easy tasks you can quickly get out of the way. But don't spend so long on the low-priority items that you never manage to reach the important ones. Take care of the essentials first.

6. *Allowing distraction to delay you.* If you're trying to work or study in a noisy, crowded environment of hustle and bustle and constant interruption, it won't be easy. Perhaps you have no choice—you have no place else to go. Okay, but learn how to

mentally shut out distractions so you can concentrate on the task at hand. Don't encourage excessive interruptions for small talk or gossip; don't encourage such interruptions to go on and on at length. If you can choose a less distracting environment, do so.

7. *Getting upset.* Some people allow their emotions to take over. They worry about their impossible load. They get angry over continual intrusions by clients or customers. They curse under their breath at the constantly ringing phone. Such tension just wastes time and energy and makes it more difficult to get done what you've got to do. Avoid unpleasant situations when possible, but when you've got no choice, just plod on as best you can on an even emotional keel.

8. *Not scheduling.* Don't let the schedule become an end in itself. But unless your memory is perfect, you'd better spend some time organizing your day, composing a list of tasks, or writing down appointments in your calendar. Otherwise, you might miss something important and screw up royally.

9. *Doing things out of a meaningful sequence.* Some tasks depend upon correct sequencing of the subtasks. Have you ever sat down to produce a poster at the last minute and suddenly realized that you had no poster board and the stores were closed? Before you get to the final stage of a project, make sure you've assembled all the materials and gotten all the input you'll need.

10. *Losing motivation.* It's tough following any of the recommendations above if you've stopped caring. From time to time, remind yourself why you're in the job, the position, or the relationship you're in. If it really doesn't make sense anymore and you see a sensible way to change, then maybe that's the solution. But if you're going to stay where you are, make the best of it.

Manage Time Better to Preserve Your Mental Health

Continually falling prey to the time busters just discussed can lead you into inefficiency, horrible stress, and wasted opportunity. It can even lead to you missing promotions or losing your job.

Conversely, learning to manage your time better can boost efficiency, help you minimize stress, and make you perform better.

Which side of this coin do you want to land on? Which will better boost your self-esteem and preserve your sanity?

CHAPTER 34

Learn to Say No

Nearly everyone recognizes the importance of saying no and would frequently like to. But many have trouble doing it, or at least doing it in a pleasant way that doesn't alienate others.

The Importance of Saying No

- *Only you can control your schedule.* People who can't turn others down end up having their days overloaded to an impossible degree. You must take charge of your life and your schedule if you want to maintain a more reasonable pace of life and accomplish the things you truly need to. The only way to assert control is by being able to turn down some of the countless demands on your time.

- *Saying no helps others grow.* If you always give in to your kids, you'll simply spoil them. They need to learn discipline and how to get along with others by not demanding everything their own way. In a group setting, active people who achieve a lot seem to get asked more and more for things. When they say no occasionally, that gives an opportunity for less active people to make their mark while learning something new.

- *Becoming more assertive helps you grow, too.* Some people feel it's a sign of compassion and generosity never to say no, to do everything that others want. While compassion may be a motive, always giving in actually indicates weakness or immaturity. Taking more control over your own time reflects psychological strength, mature judgment, positive self-esteem, and the ability to stand up for what you believe. For some, this is a slow developmental process; it doesn't just happen overnight.

How to Say No

Maintain an Assertive Stance

Mrs. K. was a high school teacher who frequently got bullied by a couple of her students. She would stand there livid, trembling, and making empty threats of reporting them to the principal. They would just laugh and mock her, knowing she didn't mean it. Many people have an instinctive ability to read others and perceive when they're serious and mean what they say. One reason is that we often subconsciously adopt a facial demeanor, a bodily posture, and a vocal quality that betray us. Our body language fairly shouts out whether we must be taken seriously or not. The good news is that you can consciously adopt the visage and demeanor of someone who means what he or she says. It's best to:

- Stand reasonably straight (but not rigid).
- Stand square in the middle of the space where you are (not leaning against a desk, wall, or doorjamb).
- Don't fidget or make distracting, repetitive, nervous moves such as tapping your toe, cracking your knuckles, or toying

with your fingernails. If you need to, hold a notebook or pencil to keep your hands occupied.

- Make frequent eye contact (but don't stare or glare).

- Speak firmly and clearly but not loudly or with obvious emotion.

- Maintain a pleasant, friendly face (but don't seem too ingratiating or eager to please).

Offer Constructive Alternatives

Negotiate with requesters who ask more of you than you want to give. Don't just turn down their concept or plan and leave them high and dry. If you can think of something appropriate, suggest another way they can accomplish their goal without you playing the role they envision. For instance:

- Agree to do part of what they ask and suggest someone else who might help with the rest.

- Confirm that you can't do the task but that you'll find someone else more willing to do it.

- Recommend another course of action for reaching the goal—one that's simpler and less time consuming.

- Suggest a less ambitious goal or a more lenient timetable for reaching it.

Once You Decide, Stay Firm

What if they don't like your alternative suggestion and persist in the original request? Occasionally, the ensuing discussion may reveal additional facts you hadn't thought of, and you honestly change your mind and now want to do whatever it is. That's okay, provided they've persuaded you with facts and logic rather than psychological manipulation. If you still feel put upon, however, and are loath to give in, don't. Remain firm. Don't let emotions or the fear of being a big blue meanie make you yield. But also don't get locked into a vicious cycle of them asking and you saying no and them simply repeating the request. Break off the encounter when it becomes obvious you're not getting anywhere with this person. Just politely excuse yourself and disappear, with your last word on the subject being that big, unambiguous *no*.

End the Encounter on a Positive Note

Hopefully, few if any of your encounters will go so badly as this. Most people, even desperate group or program chairpersons, will graciously accept a no (even if they grouse about it privately afterward). Try to confirm in their minds that you made the right decision. For instance, you can reaffirm your allegiance to the group effort and how happy you would be to help in some other way (suggest one to two that sincerely interest you). Or spell out how the additional time free of this task will help you accomplish something else (like keeping your spouse happy or taking the kids to soccer practice). Even if none of this applies, you can say something pleasant such as, "Thanks for considering me. And I hope that you find someone else." The point is not to make people feel you're rejecting them as friends or colleagues when you reject their request. Don't burn any bridges behind you—one day you may need to ask them for a favor.

CHAPTER 35

Handle Stress at Work

Adults with jobs typically spend more waking hours at work than anywhere else. Many spend more time with colleagues at the job site than with their spouses, children, other family members, and nonwork friends. Some people like it that way. As we'll see in chapter 44, some folks become workaholics because they find the structure and prescribed relationships at work more comfortable than the unpredictable and freewheeling responsibilities and demands at home.

But others find considerable conflict, tension, stress, and emotional turmoil at work. They'd rather be somewhere else—perhaps anywhere else—but can't afford to give up their jobs because they need the money. If your work environment is wonderful, then you may not find this chapter very helpful. But if any of the following work conflicts sound all too familiar, then please read on.

Typical Stresses at Work

- *Overload.* Do you have more work than you can comfortably handle? More than is humanly possible, yet it keeps on coming? Check out chapter 32 on simplifying your life, chapter 33 on managing your time, and chapter 34 on learning to say no.

- *Disruptive colleagues.* Is there someone in your group who's always on your case? Someone who drains too much of your time through continual interruptions or too much chitchat? Do you have clients or customers who are difficult, rude, demanding, or otherwise unpleasant? Please consult chapter 46 on handling problem people and chapter 51 on maintaining a positive attitude.

- *Boss problems.* Is your boss the aggressive, screamer type who likes to rule by intimidating others? Does he make stupid mistakes yet blame you when things go wrong? Is she discombobulated, ineffective, and unable to make decisions? See below.

- *Job mismatch.* Are the people at work okay, but the work just not to your liking? Do you get sick from doing the same old junk over and over again? Would you rather be doing something else but can't find an opening in that field? We'll discuss this later in this chapter.

Surviving Work Stresses

As noted just above, several previous chapters have dealt with handling people and situations that generally occur throughout our lives, both at work and elsewhere. But let's devote the remainder of this chapter to surviving those problems that are usually unique to the workplace.

Some General Thoughts

- *Realize that stress is universal.* Many of us suffer from the "grass is greener on the other side of the fence" syndrome. We need to realize that the cattle over there think it's greener on our side. Everybody has both problems and joys, both good and bad times at work. No place is perfect, so don't consider leaving just because you have some distress at work. Anywhere you go will have some distress.

- *Put stress to work for you.* Understand the value of stress. That whole stress reaction system was built in because it provides some benefit. Stress activates us, and our systems react in hardwired ways to help us handle it. Unfortunately, it's possible to overreact or react in inappropriate ways. But the mere presence of stress shouldn't prove our downfall. We can turn it to our advantage by channeling its energizing effects into the tasks at hand.

- *Keep stress levels within tolerable limits.* If you feel stress soaring out of control, remember the principles from chapter 4 on breathing to relax, and the other relaxation techniques in chapter 50. Don't try to cope with work stress by sloughing off, resorting to drugs or alcohol, or slipping into other negative and self-destructive behaviors.

Applications to Specific Situations

- *Keep the boss on your side.* Even the most abrasive boss can become bearable if you keep him or her on your side. Here's the secret how: you convert to his side. In other words, quit resisting his leadership and instead become a dependable team player. Tell him privately when you disagree, but in public support his goals for the company or group. Find out what he wants done, and do it. Look out for his interests at the office, keep him from being blindsided by problems, and do whatever you can to make him look good. Never, never demean or put him down or challenge him in a negative way in front of others. Instead, demonstrate loyalty, competence, and dedication. If you become one of his right-hand people, he'll look out for you even if he's the kind of boss who devastates plenty of others.

- *Learn to like your work if you can.* Okay, maybe in school you had your heart set on becoming an actor or artist or professional musician. But you've had your shot and you couldn't find a paying job in your preferred field, so you've had to settle for something else. You don't really enjoy sales or management or office work or whatever, but at least it pays a living wage and you feel stuck.

  As long as you choose to remain there, try to make the most of it. Read and learn more about your career field. Try to find at least some aspects that interest you and concentrate on them. To relieve the pressure, pursue your artistic (or other) interest on the side, after hours. If possible, integrate that interest area into your current job as well. For instance, if you adore art, see if your boss will let you contribute some designs as ads for the next sales promotion. This could make your current job more interesting and also possibly be the springboard into a whole new career for you somewhere down the line.

- *Try to leave if you must.* If you simply can't stand your job and see no way that this will change, then try to move up or move out. Maybe if you hang on just a little longer, you'll be able to get that promotion to a better position. Meanwhile, keep looking for work more to your liking elsewhere. Keep that hope alive.

Stress can make you sick and unhappy. But you can learn to master it, even to use it to enhance your performance. The latter approach is a whole lot better for your biological clock.

CHAPTER 36

Snooze or You Lose

Amid all the hurried rushing to get all of our daily tasks done, all that stress, who has time to get enough rest? Ah, but the secret to success in handling all those complex tasks is also the secret to feeling more energetic and younger. And it's the secret to beating the health-ravaging and aging effects of stress. What is this secret? Getting enough rest.

We know, we know . . . when you've got only seventeen waking hours in the day, there's just no time for a rest, is there? But what if a half-hour rest made it possible for you to do far more (and better) work in the sixteen and a half hours remaining than you could possibly do in seventeen while feeling exhausted and drained? Sleeping better at night and getting a twenty- to thirty-minute rest or nap period midday will do just that for you!

Sleep Better at Night

The majority of Americans suffer insomnia at least occasionally. Don't you dread that feeling of waking up even more tired than when you went to bed, feeling the life just drain out of you as you try to tackle the demands of the day while exhausted and sleepy? You don't merely feel bad, but tend to make more mistakes and risk serious danger as well. Dr. William Dement's sleep research at Stanford University found that some sleep-deprived people lapse into microsleeps of a second or two duration without warning and without realizing it. Yet the brain-wave monitors they were hooked up to revealed a brief loss of consciousness, one that could cause a serious accident if driving, for example. No wonder that a massive study of one million Americans over a six-year period, conducted by the American Cancer Society, found that people getting less than seven hours sleep a night were more likely to die during the study than those getting more.

Fortunately, there are ways to defeat insomnia.

How to Relax and Fall Asleep

- *Minimize caffeine intake.* "Impossible!" you say. "I couldn't make it through the day without my coffee!" While it's true that caffeine helps keep you awake and alert when you're trying to function, it unfortunately does the same when you're trying to sleep. It doesn't just vanish from the system at bedtime—it takes hours and hours for your body to metabolize it all. Therefore, consume as little caffeine as possible, and do it as early in the day as possible. And realize that it's not only the obvious coffee and tea that contain it, but also most colas, chocolate, and many over-the-counter medications (such as some headache remedies).

- *Avoid excitation (other than sex) two to three hours before bedtime.* Try to avoid intense exercise, worrisome work, arguments, and other stressful interactions before trying to go to sleep. It takes time for the stress hormones to subside and allow your nerves to relax.

- *Take a relaxing, warm bath an hour or two before bedtime.* Research at the Sleep Disorders Center and Sleep Research Program at McLean Hospital in Belmont, Massachusetts, found that a warm bath raises body temperature, and the gradual cooling afterward mimics the natural drop in temperature that triggers sleep. The older women in this study, all of whom were usually insomniac, had better sleep all night long following a warm bath, as opposed to one at body temperature.

- *Do something that helps you unwind for about thirty to sixty minutes before bedtime.* Make love, watch TV, listen to soft music, sit before the fire while scratching the dog, or read your kids a bedtime story. Sometimes snacks high in carbohydrates and low in protein can help by triggering neurotransmitters associated with relaxation and sleepiness (as covered in chapter 18). Dietary supplements such as the amino acid tryptophan or the hormone melatonin may also prove useful—but check with your doctor first. And avoid sleeping pills, because these increase grogginess the next day and may become habit forming.

- *Minimize sensory stimulation in the sleep area.* Keep your bedroom dark, with heavy shades or curtains. Wear a black eyepatch if you have to. Keep the room as quiet as possible or use a noise-masking machine or fan to blot out disturbing sound. Or get soft wax earplugs from the drugstore to block the noise from reaching your ears. If you have to get up in the middle of the night, use a dim night-light rather than bright light, because the brighter the light, the more aroused you'll become.

What to Do If You Wake Before You're Ready

- *Don't worry.* Don't think how desperate you feel about missing sleep or worry how tired you'll feel in the morning. Don't keep tossing and turning or try to force yourself to fall back asleep. All the above will just excite you more and make it difficult to get back to sleep.

- *Distract yourself.* If it's late and you're wide awake, this may be a good time to watch a dull TV show or read the most boring book you can find. If you're only half awake, stay quietly in bed in the dark and occupy your mind with some senseless mental game or activity such as trying to count backward from a thousand by sevens. You also might imagine turning a bunch of pegs in a board one at a time for a quarter turn per time—or just count the proverbial sheep.

Take a Midday Siesta

No matter how well you sleep at night, if you're working hard all morning, you'll probably start feeling tired by early afternoon. Most people find that a brief fifteen- to thirty-minute nap or even just a quiet period of rest can recharge their batteries, keeping them fresh until night.

Finding Time When You're Busy

- *Schedule a period for rest.* It seems you can squeeze most of your meetings, phone calls, e-mail, and mail into a busy schedule, so just plan for a rest like any other activity. Even five minutes is better than nothing, but about fifteen to thirty is optimal.

- *Put other matters aside.* True, this won't always work. If you're taking care of a sick child, for instance, you simply can't put him or her off. But you can safely ignore lesser responsibilities for just a few minutes. Let the machine pick up your phone if it rings unexpectedly during your scheduled break.

Finding a Place to Rest at Work

If you work at home or live close enough to work that you can return home for lunch, then you've got it made. Some enlightened companies have recognized the value of rest for boosting overall productivity and allow specific nap breaks; if you work there, then you've got it made, too. But what if you don't? What if you must stay at the work site for eight, ten, or even twelve hours but you feel really tired?

- *Rest in your car.* If you park in a fairly remote site to begin with, probably no one will ever realize that you're slipping away to your car for a break. If there's a lot of pedestrian traffic through the office parking area, try to find a spot only a few minutes away where you can drive for a quick park and rest. If the weather is cold, have blankets handy; if the weather is hot, try to park in a shady spot, open your windows, and/or use a portable battery-operated fan. *Don't* risk falling asleep while parked with your engine running so you can keep the heater or air conditioner on—occasionally people die that way from carbon monoxide poisoning. Carry an alarm clock to make sure you wake up in time.

- *Rest in an isolated spot in the building.* If you can't leave the building, find a quiet, remote spot where hopefully no one will find or bother you for a few minutes. For instance, is there a library or reading room with chairs in quiet corners?

- *Try the office.* If all else fails, rest in your own office at your own desk, sitting up. Close the door if you have a private office. If all you have is a cubicle, but your colleagues are supportive, then tell those nearby when you're taking your break so they'll respect your privacy; if they aren't so accommodating, turn your back to other people so they won't see that your eyes are closed. Pick a time when most people are away or there are fewer interruptions from customers, visitors, or callers. If all you have is a desk in an open room, you may be out of luck, unless you can find a quiet spot elsewhere.

If you're not comfortable falling asleep in such cases, just close your eyes, breathe deeply and slowly, relax your muscles, empty your mind of worries, and think of peaceful or relaxing scenes. If

you reach a deep state of relaxation and remain there for a few minutes, you'll feel almost as restored as if you had actually slept.
Try it and see!

For more information on getting a good night's sleep, try these Web sites:

- www.asda.org (of the American Sleep Disorders Association).

- www.sleepfoundation.org (of the National Sleep Foundation).

CHAPTER 37

Strengthen Your Memory

Have you ever heard these sayings before? "Memory is the first thing to go"; "When you get older, you can remember your twelfth birthday but not what you just had for breakfast"; "Once you lose it, you'll never get it back."

Well, there's a grain of truth behind these stereotypes: many people find their memories declining as they age. A recent survey of Americans over forty, conducted by KRC Research & Consulting, found that an estimated 144 million people may suffer from age associated memory impairment (AAMI). It doesn't have to be as bad as you may fear, though. You *can* bust this sign of age and keep your memory sharp.

How? There are all kinds of ways—behavioral tricks, mental exercises, and even diet to enhance the memory-building chemicals in your brain. But let's begin first with a brief discussion of how memory works.

How Memory Works

The exact neurophysiological and biochemical processes underlying memory are still not completely understood, but the basics go like this: The brain is composed of billions of cells called neurons. These are interconnected in a vastly complicated network and communicate with each other through chemicals known as neurotransmitters. When a new experience, sensation, or thought arises (say, hearing a new phone number), specific neurons become active. When this event is repeated or reinforced over time, new permanent links can be formed among neurons. These links are normally stored not randomly, but in meaningful patterns. For instance, your home phone number is probably stored in association with your home address, images and memories of your home, and with other phone numbers such as your office phone or fax. Thus, organized material is easier to learn than jumbled or fragmented bits of data. Before a permanent connection is made, it's very easy to forget something—for example, you hear a new name at a party but it doesn't quite register and you simply can't recall it. But after a long-term association has been structured (using chemicals provided by diet), it may never be lost (except through brain damage), and you may possibly retrieve it later even if you have difficulty doing so. Impressions made more vivid by robust motivation or emotion or inputs from several senses at once are more likely to be strongly stored and more readily retrieved. The older you get, however, the more total memories your brain holds, and the more difficult it can become to add distinct new ones. Imagine, for example, a child trying to find a toy in a closet with five toys; now imagine that same person at age seventy trying to find an item in a "closet" of five million memories.

With this understanding in mind, let's examine how memories can be enhanced at all levels of this process. Some of these rely on basic common sense, but you should realize more fully now why they work. Some are well known, yet people repeatedly fail to use them and then wonder why they keep forgetting things.

Behavioral Tricks to Enhance Memory

Employ Triggers

Triggers are reminders, things that jog your memory. Imagine, if you will, a string tied to a specific memory that enables you to pull it to consciousness at will. Try some specific reminders like these:

- *Organize material you want to learn and remember.* Keep a small pad and pen handy at all times in your pocket or purse. Make it a full-sized pocket calendar or schedule book if you're so inclined. Write down important meetings, appointments, and tasks to fulfill. Organize this information by date, topic, or whatever makes the most sense to you.

- *Associate new items to remember with fixed events.* For example, if you go golfing every Saturday but need also to go buy some aspirin next Saturday, create a mental image of yourself stopping off at the drugstore after leaving the golf course. You won't forget to play golf, but then when you get in the car afterward, the need for your pharmacy stop should pop into awareness.

- *Write notes.* Write notes for yourself or others and leave them in strategic spots near where the action will take place. For instance, write a note that you need to get gas and leave it on the driver's seat—not your night table.

- *Use multiple sensory inputs.* If you note in a newspaper the name of a new movie you want to see, for instance, say the name out loud and then imagine the smell of the popcorn in the theater.

Develop Routines

Let's say you sometimes forget to take your prescription medicine during your morning rush to get out of the house. You could use a trigger such as a note or leaving the bottle beside your hat, coat, or handbag. But you could also help by building a regular routine of taking the pill, say, when you first walk into the kitchen. If that becomes habitually your first act after turning on the light, you'll be less likely to forget it. You can build such a routine by first deciding on the best course of action—when, where, and how you'll do the specific deed. Initially, you must consciously remind yourself (or use triggers) to keep doing it every time necessary. After a few repetitions, however, you'll develop an unconscious habit that you probably won't forget.

Reduce Stress

Stress impairs memory, while extreme stress or panic makes it virtually impossible to remember much at all. If stress is interfering with memory formation, learn to reduce the stress first. See chapter 4 on relaxed breathing and chapter 50 on progressive relaxation techniques, for more details.

Mental Exercises to Enhance Memory

Concentrate

Dividing your attention too many ways robs you of the ability to store the memory properly in the first place. There are so many neural circuits active at once that the brain can't decide what to store and where to store it. You're not really forgetting so much as ignoring the information from the start, an all-too-common problem in this day and age. For the unimportant details of life, this doesn't matter. For something important—like the name of a new client—learn to turn off other concerns and focus on the information when you first hear it. Repeat it silently to yourself a few times. This provides your brain the clarity to make the right connection.

Practice, Practice, Practice

Just like any other skill, your memory can use some practice. Tend to forget the names of your friends' kids? Make a written list and train your memory by testing yourself, just as if you were back in fifth grade learning state capital names. You'll probably find that you learn and remember just as well as when you were ten—provided you practice. In addition to rehearsing specific items you want to remember, exercise your memory in general by daily doing some memory-requiring task like a crossword puzzle or trivia game.

Expect Positive Results

Don't ever tell yourself, "I'll never remember all that." And don't label yourself as a forgetter, someone with a problem memory. Such negative expectations produce self-fulfilling prophecies and your memory may fail—but for artificial reasons rather than aging. Instead, encourage yourself. Tell yourself you will remember to greet your boss's spouse by name at the party that evening. Expect the memory to pop up when needed, and more often than not it will.

Create Vivid Visual Associations

What if you suddenly remember something important but don't have a pad handy? Make up an unusual mental picture that will stick with you. For instance, you suddenly recall that you forgot to buy vitamins and apples in your last shopping trip. Envision something wild that links these two items—say, an image of a giant smiling, walking apple with a hat made of an enormous purple and pink polka-dot vitamin pill. You won't be able to forget something like that even if you try!

Using Diet to Enhance Memory

We know that the brain stores memories chemically in its neurons. This process depends upon both protein to make the structural changes and, in addition to others, a chemical called acetylcholine to facilitate signal transmission among memory cells. Thus, a diet severely deficient in either protein (see chapter 5 for ideas on protein sources such as meat, cheese, and beans) or choline (the starting point for acetylcholine) can disrupt memory and intellectual functioning (see below). Ditto for the B vitamins (see chapter 17). This doesn't mean, however, that gorging on these nutrients will give you a super memory. You need enough of both, *but not an excess.*

Let's talk now about some of the ordinary foods that contain choline and should be a regular part of your diet. These include wheat germ, egg yolks, lentils, nuts, liver, cabbage, and cauliflower. There's also a choline-containing food additive called lecithin that's found in a wide variety of processed foods.

Recipes to Help Keep Memory Sharp

How's this for a memory-enhancing breakfast?

- Cold cereal, any type low in sugar, with low-fat milk and covered with several tablespoons of wheat germ.

- One egg prepared according to choice. (Remember not to eat more than four eggs per week due to the fat and cholesterol.)

- A small bowl of lentils, spiced to taste (more on lentils and lentil preparation in chapter 11).

Then, for your midmorning snack, have a small one-once packet of nuts. Don't overdo nuts, because they contain lots of fat as well as their protein. In fact, go for the leaner, low-fat sources of protein when possible.

What About Herbs?

Some people take herbs such as ginkgo biloba to improve memory. Some research supports this notion, while other studies don't. See chapter 18 for more details.

CHAPTER 38

Become More Creative

When you were a kid, you couldn't wait to get out of school so you could go play. You'd spend hours with your friends and your toys playing out all sorts of pretend situations. Your daydreams were rich and unlimited. Your imagination seemed boundless. If you're like most of us, you began to lose a lot of that creativity as you grew up. You started getting into a rut, into habits and routines that limited the scope of your vision. Perhaps your employer rejected many of your creative ideas and wanted you to do things his or her way. Perhaps the multiple demands of job, family, and continued training left you too exhausted to think. Far from anticipating a bright future, you were grateful and relieved merely to have survived yet one more day of the present. Eventually, your creative thought became limited to such decisions as whether you should channel-surf up or down the scale this time.

But don't give up. You can regain some of that lost spark of creativity and vivid imagination. You can break out of your routine to grow more mentally sharp, younger, and happier. You can become more creative at work, at home, and in your relationships.

Tap Into Your Creativity

If you're motivated enough to be reading this book, then you're certainly bright enough to have a wellspring of creative ideas. If you don't feel that way right now, it's probably because you've deliberately and habitually suppressed the creative child within you. The best way to break through such barriers and wake him or her back up is to brainstorm, either with others or by yourself. Here's how:

- *Listen to your subconscious.* Too often we turn a deaf ear to our own ideas. They start to bubble up and we, in essence, shout at them, "Shut up! I'm too busy right now!" Often they will pop out again when our conscious mind isn't so vigilant, such as when we're relaxing, falling asleep, dreaming, or first awakening. Practice trying to listen at such times, trying to coax the idea into full consciousness.

- *Jot down all ideas.* Good ideas have a habit of disappearing quickly as we dart to and fro in the hubbub of daily life. Write them down at once so you won't forget. Keep paper and a pen or pencil with you at all times practicable—perhaps on your person, beside your bed, and in your car. What if you get fantastic ideas when in the shower, where writing isn't very practical? Just keep rehearsing the idea mentally until you can wrap up the shower quickly and write it down.

- *Organize and interrelate ideas.* Once you write them down, store or file them in an organized way. For instance, assemble all your notes for a new project together. Keep this pile or file separate from the one on that new poem you want to write or that surprise birthday party you're planning. Periodically look over the file to see how the ideas connect or mutually build upon one another.

- *Don't criticize your ideas too soon.* Self-editing of an idea or criticism by others too soon effectively kills it. Don't do that.

Let it percolate a while and it might lead you to another, better idea, even if you eventually reject this first one.

- *Discuss your concepts.* This is the heart of group brainstorming. But even if you've been brainstorming by yourself, there comes a point where you need to bounce your concepts off someone else. Discuss your thoughts with your spouse, other relatives, or close friends. Their comments may stimulate you into new directions, over obstacles you had run into, and their support may encourage you to continue.

- *Evaluate and prioritize.* You probably won't have time or money to put into effect all your ideas, no matter how good they are. Develop some kind of sorting scheme to figure out which are your best ideas—the ones you want to try to implement first. Maybe you'll have time for the others later. But if not, work through your best, most important stuff first.

Apply Creativity to All Areas of Life

Become More Creative at Work

Brainstorming as just described can be immensely helpful at work. Yes, your boss may occasionally shoot down your ideas. But she'll probably respect and value you more because you're at least producing ideas rather than just blindly trudging down the treadmill. She'll see your potential. The next step is to get more in tune with her goals and plans for the office so that you'll develop ideas more relevant in her eyes.

Become More Creative at Home

We don't advocate making changes just for the sake of change or proving you can "be spontaneous" by plunging into something without thinking about it. On the other hand, don't stay in ruts just out of habit. Look with fresh eyes at how you've laid out the furniture, organized your possessions, or decorated your home. Can you think of some approach that's not merely different or novel but might actually improve things? Discuss it first with the others who might be affected by such a change, and then try it out. You can always go back to the familiar if it doesn't work out.

Become More Creative in Your Relationships

We know a couple who try to outdo each other in coming up with wonderfully creative ways to celebrate key events such as anniversaries and birthdays. One time she might develop a Hawaiian theme, with clothes, decorations, and dinner to match. Another time he might surprise her with tickets to an audience participation mystery theater, where they can join with the actors in trying to solve a pretend murder mystery. While some couples like to celebrate by trying new places and activities, others prefer tradition and return to the scene of their honeymoon on every anniversary. Becoming more creative doesn't mean you have to shake up every area of your life and shed all tradition. In such cases, apply creativity by making your own anniversary cards, selecting special gifts, or expressing love in novel ways. There's a place for both comfortable habit and creative spontaneity in all human relationships.

Becoming more creative will make you feel—and appear—more alive and vital. And this renewal of your mind will help slow your biological clock.

CHAPTER 39

Listen to the Music

"**M**usic hath charms to soothe the savage breast," as the old saying goes. Knowing the power of music to alter our minds and emotions, merchandisers use music in advertising jingles or as background sound, politicians use it to stir the voters in campaigns, and some employers use it to keep workers docile and content. And of course, what would be the emotional impact of a movie without accompanying music?

Music is entwined with all aspects of our lives. It writes itself indelibly on our memories, attaching to the highs and lows, the sweet and bitter moments of our fleeting hours. Isn't there a special song that you associate with a standout first date or your wedding? Hearing that song years later may carry you back on wings of remembrance to that intimate and meaningful time. You don't merely recall it . . . you go back there and relive it. You savor again the emotions, the images, the sensations of the whole experience.

If music has such potency, there should be no surprise that we can harness its horsepower in the drive to slow our biological clocks.

The Many Benefits of Music

- *Relaxation.* After a tough day at work, turn on the radio or stereo to some soothing music. It'll help you unwind from the rigors of the day and restore your mental and emotional equilibrium.

- *Stimulating creativity.* Great music inspires you. It unleashes intellectual and creative juices. If you're working on an original project, whether writing a poem or a work report, and reach a mental block, play some of your favorite music. Things will start bubbling up in your mind, and you'll probably find your solution.

- *Enhancing mood.* Sometimes, even if you're relaxed, you may feel blah. Sorta down. Kinda blue. Listen to some good music with an upbeat tempo. Better yet, move to the music—tap your foot or even dance. The blues will fly away with the beat.

- *Improving health.* Tranquil music reduces tension, stress, and high blood pressure. This isn't just a placebo effect involving self-deception, either, because even some animals react better during good music. You don't just feel better emotionally, you actually measure better on physiological tests. For instance, research in the music therapy program at Appalachian State found that after listening to classical music for six weeks, all the subjects in the study not only self-reported less fatigue and depression, but had objectively lower levels of stress hormones in their bloodstreams.

So if you ever feel about to explode from the pressure on your life, turn to pleasant music. It could help save your life! Better music than a stress heart attack.

Choosing the Right Music

All music is not created equal.
Music is a tool that can be used for bad as well as good. If some

music can exalt your imagination and spirit, other music can de-
press, terrify, or otherwise upset you. Its emotional power may
tend to overpower your rational mind and lead you into stupid,
dangerous, or other maladaptive behavior. It can affect you physically. The eerie music in a horror movie, for instance, can send
your blood pressure and heart rate soaring.

One Person's Music Is Another Person's Noise

There is clearly a generation gap in music appreciation. Each
younger generation usually adopts a style that shocks its parents.
(On the other hand, nostalgic resurgences of old music may attract
young listeners, too.) Even within the same generation, tastes vary
widely. Some prefer classical, others pop. The same piece of music
that elevates one person's mood may turn someone else cold.

Music With Melody and Harmony Beats Raucous Junk

Irrespective of what tastes people may adopt from mere exposure over time or peer pressure, certain kinds of music usually
have fixed effects. Here's a couple of obvious examples:

- Which music would you associate with being serene and relaxed—classical symphony or heavy metal?

- Which music would you associate with being keyed up,
  angry, aggressive, and antisocial—soft pop or acid rock?

Aren't the answers obvious? Even some animals respond differently to such extremes in music. Be aware of these differences and
use them wisely. People who like heavy metal don't find it inspiring
and relaxing in the same way as others who prefer Bach and other
classical composers. The metalheads apparently desire to have
their systems churned inside out by the wild stuff. Not a good idea
in our book—not if you want to slow your biological clock.

CHAPTER 40

Hop on the Reading Railroad

Some people actually brag that they've never read a book since high school. To them, reading was an awful chore forced on them by a dreaded educational establishment. Graduating was like finishing a prison term. They weren't about to do any of "that reading stuff" once they were free!

You might just as well be glad for "freedom" from intelligence, wisdom, clear thinking, memory, emotional balance, spiritual insight, and even good health. These are the kinds of benefits reading helps bestow.

The Benefits of Good Reading

Enhance Your Mental Abilities

Like your muscles, your brain needs regular exercise to stay strong. Any kind of active learning helps, not only that involving reading. But the written word provides many more opportunities and more ready availability than such other avenues as audio training, video training, internships, and so on. Reading opens the whole universe and all of history and philosophy to you. It expands your consciousness, sharpens your intellect, adds to your store of facts and wisdom, and strengthens your logical skills. Research has demonstrated that much of the mental decline often associated with aging stems from voluntary disuse rather than inevitable aging per se. This means that people who stop using their minds do begin to lose them as they grow older. But people who strive to keep mentally active and alert throughout life keep their brain cells more vibrant and alive. Reaction time is faster, memory is quicker and more complete, logic is more accurate. Do you want your mind to turn to mush as you grow older or to keep humming along like a fine watch? Regular reading can really help make the difference.

Illuminate Your Emotional, Psychological, and Spiritual Life

It's been said that the unexamined life is not worth living. As you grow older, it becomes more important to see the big picture and how you and your life fit in. Scripture helps provide a moral framework and a philosophical viewpoint that can contribute meaning and purpose to your life. Reading nonfiction such as history and biography helps keep you in tune with the nature of humanity. Great fiction that clarifies the inner workings of the mind can shed light on your own psyche.

Provide a Solid Foundation for Health

The very fact that you're reading this book perfectly illustrates this point. By keeping up with the latest developments in medicine, exercise, nutrition, psychology, and so on, you're learning concepts that can add years or even decades to your life. The odds are that you enjoy greater health than your parents (and almost certainly than your grandparents) did at your age now. Part of this flows from scientific advances in the fields just cited—but only by staying abreast of them can you fully derive their benefits. What good is it to you if we have new herbal remedies for depression, foods with better nutrition, or innovative techniques for early self-detection of deadly diseases if you remain unaware of them and never use them? Keep reading!

How to Read

Have you ever read when tired or otherwise distracted, gone line by line down a whole page, started to turn the page, and suddenly realized that you hadn't absorbed a single word? Like a car revving in neutral, your body parts went through the motions, but your brain wasn't in gear. If you're just reading something light for pure recreation, this doesn't matter. But if you're reading something serious from which you wish to benefit by more than simple relaxation, you need to concentrate.

Find Time to Read

Stay in tune with reality by keeping up with current events. Read a newspaper, news magazine, or newsletter just about every day. If you don't have time to read it all at once, that's okay. Read one minute here, five minutes there; over the course of the day, you'll be able to get the highlights in.

Read lighter material when you want to relax. As you're nodding off in bed is not the best time to read a deep philosophical treatise involving intense thought. But it might be the perfect time for some light humor.

On non–work days, set aside at least an hour for some serious or catch-up reading. On a vacation, holiday, or bad-weather day, maybe you can squeeze in even more time. There's nothing like being snowbound or rained in and curling up with a good book by the fire.

Read for life in both senses of the phrase. That is, keep reading all your life. When you stop moving forward, you start falling behind. And read for the purpose of enhancing your life, bettering your physical and mental health, busting the signs of age. It works!

CHAPTER 41

Travel to Tranquillity

Sometimes you really, really need a vacation. Often you may feel like just vegging out at home or at some familiar spot. But we suggest that once in a while you try something new, original, or different. Go to a place you've never been before, perhaps try something daring. If you can afford it, go far away, perhaps someplace where they don't speak your language, where the people, the customs, the money, the food are all very different. Go rock climbing in Norway, skiing in the South American Andes, or snorkeling in Bermuda. If all these sound too strenuous, then just head for a resort or spa where you can relax and feel pampered for a while. You know what you like, so go for it!

Enjoy These Benefits of Travel

Done right, all travel can restore you, providing fun and exhilaration. But let's focus here on travel to new (to you) or exotic locations.

Break Out of Your Box

Travel takes you out of your routine—not only your work cycle but also your habitual way of looking at life. It challenges and rein-

vigorates your mind. And you'll be astonished how quickly in a foreign country you pick up the basic words you need to get by and
get used to the local currency without having to convert it into dollars mentally. You'll adapt to—and enjoy—the manners and ways
of the local people.

Gain a Fresh Perspective

Becoming familiar with a new culture makes you more aware of
the diversity of human life. You begin to better understand the
cross-cultural conflicts that underlie many contemporary global
developments and current news events. It also helps provide a new
perspective on the strengths and weaknesses of your own culture.
For example, you may decide that you prefer the slower pace of
life often seen in Europe or Latin America and gain a fresh resolve
to loaf a bit more when you return home.

Develop Empathy

Empathy, the ability to understand and feel for others, is part of
what makes us human. Visiting other cultures increases empathy
by providing first-hand knowledge of what foreigners talk, think,
and care about. As long as people from Country X remain strangers,
they seem strange. Once you visit, see them, and perhaps make
friends, they no longer appear so different. You perceive the commonality among all people and come to better appreciate such dis-
parities as do exist.

Feel Young Again

Enjoying new experiences, as long as you don't obsess about it,
energizes you, builds self-confidence, and boosts self-esteem. The
break from routine gives you more zest for living and restores your
psychological balance. You look and feel younger during and after
an exciting travel vacation.

Tips for Safe and Healthy Travel

Don't Overdo It

Traveling at a reasonable rate can provide the many benefits cited above. But if you force a frenzied pace and try to do everything you can possibly cram into each twenty-four-hour period, you may simply exhaust yourself. Listen to your body and rest when you need to. Better to bypass that "one more" museum or nightspot than to wear yourself out to the point that you're not so much enjoying sights as aggressively ticking off a checklist of required duties.

Maintain Security

Nothing ruins a vacation like losing your money or falling victim to crime. Police departments and the U.S. State Department, among others, provide extensive information on the keys to security and safety. But really it boils down to alertness, common sense, and trusting your instincts. For example, don't become an obvious target in public by showing large quantities of cash, talking about money, or leaving valuables such as purses and wallets where they can be easily seen and snatched. Use traveler's checks or credit cards rather than carry excess cash. Keep return tickets and other valuables in a hotel safe or other locked and secure spot. If a location looks sleazy and starts ringing alarm bells in your mind, pay heed—don't go there!

Bring Essentials With You

Depending upon where you're going and whom you're traveling with, you may need to bring a lot of essentials with you. This applies particularly to items such as spare eyeglasses or prescription medicines. Don't assume you can refill a prescription anywhere; bring enough for your entire stay and a slight reserve in case your return is delayed. If you wear a MediAlert bracelet or have any special medical conditions that could possibly flare up without warning, try to get that vital medical information translated into the languages of the countries you plan to visit. Print it on a ready carry card *before you leave home.*

Maintain an Upbeat Attitude

Every trip has its share of little disasters. Later, they will make some of your most interesting, amusing, and memorable anecdotes. For instance, years ago Charles visited Mont-Saint-Michel on the coast of France with friends. They all missed the last bus out and had to walk to the nearest town, where they couldn't find a hotel vacancy anywhere. The train station was closed for the night and there was no way to get to the next town. They spent the night huddled together in a park, freezing and unable to sleep. This became the most vivid and unforgettable day of the trip.

Later you'll enjoy talking about such incidents. So while they're happening, you may as well take that future perspective and try to accept them now as just another part of your adventure. You may not actually enjoy struggling through a mishap, but if you remain upbeat you'll certainly pull through it better. You'll be more alert to possible solutions to your problem. And a little humor at such times can alleviate a lot of the anxiety or distress.

PART V

Work Toward Delightful Relationships

To someone who's constantly lonely, using exercise and nutrition and so on to improve health and longevity may seem pointless. Some may feel that if life is unsatisfying, why want more of it? So to fully consider ways to bust your age, we turn now to the beauties and joys and benefits of relationships, and later in part 6 to other ways to enhance emotional well-being. Having close-knit, warm relationships boosts health and happiness; it also provides a major incentive for taking care of yourself in other ways.

CHAPTER 42

Rekindle the Romance

Individuals who are happily married tend to feel better about themselves. They're healthier both physically and emotionally. According to Linda Waite of the sociology department at the University of Chicago, they have sex more often and enjoy it more. A major study of eighteen thousand adults in seventeen different advanced nations found that married people generally have higher levels of health and overall happiness as well as financial stability. They get more out of life and live longer, too!

Not every couple is happily married, of course. With lives growing busier and more stress filled, many couples drift away from each other over time. They end up feeling lonely or embittered within the marriage and seek divorce in hopes of ending the misery.

Wouldn't it be wonderful if two people who start off in a loving, committed relationship could remain that way forever?

They can! It's not just a matter of chance or fate. Both successful and divorcing couples on average have the same basic types and numbers of disagreements and problems. The difference comes in how they respond. Successful couples work at their relationships. And one of the best ways to keep that happy spark alive is to rekindle your sense of romance.

First, Get Your Head Straight

Realize Things Will Always Change

Some say, "That would be easy if he/she were as attentive and considerate and young looking as before. Why can't things just stay the same?" Because they can't. Wishing for a past that won't return will not help you survive the present or prepare for a brighter future. Things will change whether you want them to or not. The times—the attitudes and social pressures—change. We all change physically. Our interests and concerns evolve over time so that things once very important to us now seem trivial or meaningless, and some things we once rarely thought about now preoccupy us. Our activities and associates change as we move on to other jobs, other places to live, other organizations. We gain—and lose—family, friends, and other supporting relationships.

Learn to accept and deal with the inevitable changes that come your way.

Look for Love Inside—Not Outside—the Relationship

Many people respond to change by losing interest in the person they once loved and trying to rekindle the old feelings with someone else. They may choose someone who reminds them of how their spouse used to be. They've drifted apart, so now they want intimacy with a fresh face. What they don't seem to realize is that the new person isn't perfect either and will also change over time, like everyone else. They've based their decision to cheat or divorce on myths and fantasies taught through a thousand fictional movies, books, stories, and songs.

But reality has a way of catching up with them and biting them in the rear. Looking for love on the outside will almost certainly kill the existing relationship.

But recommitting yourself to looking for love only within the relationship is the first step toward rekindling the romance.

Second, Take Action

Make Time for Each Other

To heat up the romantic thermometer, you've got to spend time together.

* *Schedule special and regular times with each other.* Since our first year of marriage twenty-nine years ago, we've tried to celebrate our "monthiversary" every month on the numeric date of our wedding, either by going out to eat or bringing takeout home. Spend time together every day, even if it's just while cleaning up after dinner or making lunches for the next day.

* *Communicate, communicate, communicate.* When one of us is out of town on a trip, we always communicate by phone or e-mail at least once a day. Talk out issues, disagreements, and other concerns or they'll bubble up inside you until they burst through. Talk about your daily activities, your hopes and goals, what you want to do when you retire—anything and everything. Leave loving notes for each other. Even a grocery list can be transformed into a loving note if you sign off, "Thanks, love you, honey," or something similar. Communication is the lifeblood of romance.

Develop Joint Interests

It's fine for each partner to have some interests not shared by the other. People also need some time alone, a little "space" now and then. But if you have no major joint interests at all, the relationship is headed for trouble. While physical attraction may have been one of the dominant forces initially bringing you together, it won't keep you together for a lifetime all by itself.

* Join some of the same organizations—whether professional, church, or community. Attend meetings together when possible.

- Volunteer to do certain tasks together—whether serving on an organizational committee or just building your son's new bicycle from the 101 parts in the box.

- Share in each other's hobbies or special interests, as long as you don't overdo it (see the discussion of "space," above). Okay. She likes golf and he's a coin collector. Once in a while, he should join her on the links or when watching golf on TV. She can attend a regional coin show with him now and then.

- Develop common goals and work toward them. What about your next summer vacation? Talk about your possibilities, develop a joint dream, pore over brochures and ads, establish a separate savings account and congratulate each other on adding scrounged cash to it.

Do Romantic Things

Don't wait until you feel more romantic to act more romantic. Start acting that way and the feelings will follow. Psychologists have developed the term *cognitive dissonance* to explain how people change when attitudes and behavior don't match. That's dissonant. To become consistent or consonant, we can either change the attitude to match the behavior, or we can change the behavior to match the attitude. The former path to resolution is more common. Research shows that if you can induce someone to change his or her behavior, then usually the attitudes or feelings change to match the new conduct. Thus, if you gradually develop the habit of ignoring each other, your feelings will change toward not caring about each other as much. Conversely, if you consciously force yourself to act romantic, your emotional responses will soon change in a warmer, more loving direction.

Here are some examples to get you started:

- Compliment each other—on appearance, behavior, new clothes, on job success, on a meal well made, and so on.

- Hug and kiss each other—every day, without fail.

- Say you love each other—frequently and with real meaning.

- Hold hands sometimes when you walk or sit near each other.

- Talk cheerfully about your loved one to others.

- Express concern for each other. Ask about her day. If he's upset, ask why; let him talk it out. Offer to help each other.

- Say tender loving things during quiet moments alone.

- Do something sweet and unexpected now and then. Take the children out for several hours to give your spouse a rest.

- Make love. Notice we didn't say simply, "Have sex." There's a difference. A really big difference. And keep your sexual relationship private—it's the only thing that a couple share exclusively with each other. (More on blissful sex in chapter 43.)

Learn to Forgive

If you're having trouble making yourself act in a more loving fashion, the problem may be resentment over real or imagined grievances. The other person ignored you, hurt your feelings, or in some other way upset you. You're angry and don't want to feel closer to your partner.

This can be a serious problem, and there's no easy way around it. If you're very upset, probably the best thing to do next is to put some space between you for a while and try to distract yourself and cool down. Once you believe you can talk about the issue rationally, try to approach the other person and discuss the problem. Realize that in most cases the other person wasn't trying to hurt you but rather made a mistake—as all of us do from time to time. Apologize for your own past transgressions and accept an apology gracefully if it's offered. Either way, try to let it go at that point and just forgive the other person.

Paying attention to and loving someone in a committed relationship draws him or her closer to you. That little spark you bring to your romance will grow into a warm, cozy flame that will help see you through the frosts and chilly breezes of life.

CHAPTER 43

Experience Sex That Satisfies

Sex can be conducted at a purely biological level, without engaging the mind, spirit, and emotions. That may be pleasurable to a degree, but it's not ultimately satisfying. In fact, simple mechanical sex can leave some people feeling quite dissatisfied, upset, or distinctly depressed. Psychiatrists have coined the term *postcoital triste* for the kind of sadness or melancholy some people experience after such sex.

So the key to truly satisfying sex is to unite all aspects of your personality—not just the physical—with a special other person to whom you're deeply committed. Sex without love is just sex, but sex in a genuine love relationship is liberating, expansive, and satisfying. Anything less is a pale imitation.

Sweet Secrets of Sex Missed by Many People Today

Unfortunately, with today's hectic schedules, chronic exhaustion, and fragmented relationships, many people miss out on the ultimate mysteries of unifying sex. In fact, about a third of American adults have some form of sexual dysfunction—everything from lack of desire to inability to experience climax during sexual activity. This one short chapter is no substitute for sexual therapy for people with genuine medical problems or unresolved psychological issues. But the following hints can point the way to better, more fulfilling sex:

- *Feel, and express, love and concern for the other person.* With a lot of sex these days, each person is really expressing only self-love and is using the other person as an object. You know this is happening if you care only about what you're getting out of a relationship. You've transcended self when you truly care about the other person and want to fulfill his or her needs as well. But don't just feel love—express it. Tell and show the other person your love.

- *Don't criticize or reject.* This is never a good idea in a close relationship. But especially during intimate moments, don't communicate any form of disapproval or negativity to the other person. Nothing kills romantic feelings or sexual ardor faster! During sexual foreplay is no time to comment on the other person gaining weight or getting out of shape or looking older or having any other physical or personality flaws.

- *Be honest, open, free.* Get to know your beloved and let him or her get to know you. This implies talking, sharing, and spending time together in countless ways besides the bedroom, as discussed further in chapter 42 on romance. As each partner gets to know the other better over the years, each can better sense the other's needs and fulfill them. But don't just expect the other person magically to intuit your desires. Be open and free about discussing them.

- *Give and receive trust.* It certainly helps in feeling free to discuss things openly and expressing yourself sexually if you can trust the other person. Commit yourself to your partner with every fiber of your being. Prove yourself trustworthy by respecting and responding to the things he or she tells you.

And make clear that you trust your partner, provided he or she hasn't done something untrustworthy. (Here's where the ugly consequences of infidelity loom large and threaten the stability of a relationship.)

- *Don't rush.* Romance and good sex take time. If one partner tries to rush through it, that demonstrates lack of concern for the other partner. Further, romance and sex need to be deeply woven into the entire fabric of the relationship, not just occasional parts of it.

- *Develop a long-term orientation.* When you commit to love someone for life, it's easier to trust, to be yourself honestly, and to give of yourself freely. You know you're constantly building toward a brighter future.

- *Experiment.* Don't get into a rut. Be innovative, but in a warm, encouraging way. Don't try something that would shock, offend, hurt, or dehumanize the other person. If you suggest something new and find a reluctance to try it, don't demand an explanation or try to argue. Just respect your lover's feelings and move on to something else.

- *Express appreciation.* Tell your beloved afterward how wonderful it was or how thrilling he or she was.

The Physical and Mental Health Benefits of Sex

If satisfying sex is already so wonderful, you might be wondering, "Who needs any other benefits besides that?" Maybe you don't need them, but you'll get them:

- *Making love brings the two of you closer together.* The sexual relationship is the only thing typically that a couple share solely with each other, making them closer even than the dearest of friends and other relatives.

- *Love boosts happiness and life satisfaction.* It makes you more content, emotionally balanced, and satisfied with life.

- *Married couples have better health and live longer.* This has been well documented in numerous scientific studies. Some experts estimate that a good marriage can add five years to your life on the average.

There are two fundamentally different roads you can take. You can cruise down Highway Self alone, basically me-oriented, occasionally bumping into and using strangers, experiencing a lot of frustration and dissatisfaction even in sex.

Or you can zoom down Interstate Love with a we-orientation, developing a long-term and committed relationship with that one special other person, experiencing deep and meaningful sex that grows ever greater and more beautiful over time.

You've got the choice. Which road are you taking now? Is it time to change directions?

CHAPTER 44

Build A Rewarding Family Life

It's often said that none of us on our deathbed ever wishes we'd spent more time at work. Instead, we often regret not spending more time with loved ones. Yet in the hustle and bustle of daily life, too many people have no energy left at the end of the day to enjoy simply relaxing and conversing with their families. Then there are the workaholics who, though they may regret it later, often use work as an excuse to deliberately avoid spending more time at home. To them work seems more predictable, more controllable, even more comfortable than the complexities inherent in intimate relations. Instead of waiting until your final days to evaluate what you've missed at home and to effect reconciliation in strained relationships, start working through these issues now. Without delay. Discover how rewarding family life can be.

The Benefits of a Close Family

A warm, intimate family provides innumerable psychological and even physical rewards. Among these are:

- *A sense of belonging.* Everyone likes to be a part of some human unit or group that's somehow larger and more significant than themselves alone. If children don't find that sense of connectedness at home, they'll seek it in wayward peer groups that tend to lead them astray or even in criminal gangs. In a secure, close family, on the other hand, all members of all the generations still alive feel a part of something special and wonderful, something unique to be proud of. Every member, from the youngest newborn to the most senior great-grandparent, senses the cohesion, the unity, the togetherness of this wonderful and important thing called *family*.

- *Acceptance.* We all feel flawed and inferior in many ways. We all experience countless rejections in the outside world. But in a healthy, wholesome family, all members deeply sense that they're accepted despite their imperfections. Yes, the spouses sometimes argue. Yes, the parents must occasionally discipline the children. But after the anger and hurt pass, there remains the deep and abiding sense of acceptance.

- *Love.* Everyone wants love. Many look for it desperately. If you're blessed to have an affectionate family, you'll experience and enjoy this marvelous, powerful force.

- *Physical and mental health.* Experiencing love and acceptance at home provides a secure foundation to help you sustain daily stresses without being knocked out of the ring. People with a happy home life engage in fewer risk behaviors, remain healthier both mentally and physically, and tend to live years longer than others.

Strengthen Your Family Life

If all the virtues of family life are so readily apparent, why do we so often neglect this most important of human relationships? Because the blessings of a happy family don't just happen automatically: you must work for them, sacrifice for them, at times suffer for them. Words like this scare many moderns away. They want something simple, effortless, cost-free, and quick. But you can't build a solid family foundation that way. It can't be done.

Devote Time to Family

No farmer would expect to ignore his or her garden all year and still reap a bumper crop during harvest. Just so, we must spend time on our family relationships if we expect them to grow. How much time? It's impossible to say. You can't simply schedule it a month in advance as if it were an appointment. When a need requiring time arises, you must try as best you can to meet it. You won't always succeed, but try.

Give of Yourself

Be as open and honest with your family members as you can. If you make a promise, keep it. Love, cherish, help, and encourage each other. Share. Look out for the interests of your family members. Try to build each other up. If all this requires some sacrifice, make it.

Display Love and Affection

It's not enough just to feel love, though that should be there, too. Display it. Greet each family member first thing every morning. Hug each member at least once a day. Kiss your spouse. When the children are younger, kiss them, too, and tuck them into bed at night. Read to them. Teach them about life.

Another way to show people you treasure them is to keep photos of them on display in your home or at the office, and keep photos in your wallet or purse.

Give and Receive Forgiveness

Don't beat yourself up over every little failure to love your family as you should. When appropriate, apologize and ask for forgiveness. Resolve to do better next time. As you receive forgiveness, also give it. They aren't always perfect, just as you aren't.

Let your family know how much you enjoy them and appreciate them. Tell them you're proud of them and happy to be in the same family with them. When you work to make family life more uplifting and enjoyable for them, you'll find that your family has become more rewarding and satisfying for you as well.

CHAPTER 45

Become A Friend

People aren't born with friends. You must make friends, and certainly there are many advantages to doing so.

The Many Blessings of Having Friends

Emotional Gratification

People just naturally need each other; it's part of our make-up. We want someone to share life with, to talk to, to ease the pain of loneliness, grief, or other misfortune. Haven't you ever felt really down after a personal setback or a rough week, then gone out for an evening with friends and found tremendous emotional release? It turned your mood completely around.

Psychological Well-Being

People who lack friends, even if they have a close family, have limited opportunities to fulfill these emotional needs. They're less able to withstand psychological stress, and they recover more slowly from mishaps. They lack much of the joy in living that others consider ordinary. In extreme cases, they begin to feel left out, alone, isolated. Over time without human solace, they may turn into loners and develop psychological imbalances. The lack of social support provided by friends may be one factor in many psychological breakdowns.

One fascinating study found that it actually requires more mental energy to ignore people than to relate to them. Kristin Sommer at Baruch College in New York found that subjects who worked on word puzzles in the same room as a stranger did worse on the puzzles when they tried to ignore the stranger than when they were told to make small talk (but not share puzzle solutions) with them. It was harder on them psychologically to stay apart than to socialize.

Enhanced Health

If friends can have such profound effects on the mind, it should come as no surprise that they enhance physical health also. People with warm, satisfying friendships tend to have:

- Lower blood pressure and less risk of circulatory disease. For example, a Swedish study reported in the *European Heart Journal* found that among women hospitalized for heart problems, those with the most friends had the least severe arterial clogging.
- More resistance to stress-related disorders.
- Enhanced immunity, which in turn helps in resisting all infectious diseases. For instance, a study at Carnegie Mellon University found that when adults were exposed to a cold virus, those with the strongest network of friends got the least sick, while those with fewer friends developed more cold symptoms.

This doesn't mean, of course, that having a friend ensures a lifetime of perfect health. But it does mean that you boost your chances of health compared to those who are lonely and miserable.

How to Make Friends

To win a friend, you must become a friend. To attract others, you must prove yourself friendly. Here are some basic tips:

- *Listen to others.* Imagine that you try to share something really personal, and it soon becomes obvious that the other person hasn't heard a single word. Now reverse positions. If you want to prove you're a friend, actively listen to others when they try to tell you something. Drop whatever else you're concentrating on and focus on them. Make them feel special, respected, cared for. They will instantly pick up on your display of friendliness and be more likely to respond in kind.

- *Share others' interests.* People with dissimilar work lives, community activities, and recreational interests will have little to talk about, to share, and aren't likely to become friends unless there's some other area of commonality to bind them, such as living next door. The more interests, beliefs, and activities two people have in common, the more likely they are to want to be together and to become friends. You can make use of this principle by deliberately exploring the interest area of someone with whom you'd like to become friendly. Who knows, maybe the stamp collector will find that he actually likes watching basketball if he gives it a chance.

- *Don't criticize.* A friendship is rewarding because each partner provides affirmation and positive "strokes" to the other. But criticism is a negative stroke that rapidly drives others away. One bitter criticism can wipe out the positive impression of a hundred earlier warm comments. Don't do it, not ever, if you want to remain friends. There may be times when you feel the other person is about to make a huge mistake or take a terrible misturn in life. At such times, you may feel compelled to try to help. Okay, but do it in a loving, respectful way by helping your friend explore the possible implications of a decision. Simply barking critical, judgmental, or negative comments does *not* help in such cases.

• *Don't give advice unless asked.* Unsolicited advice is often considered as a criticism and merely annoys most people. Even if asked, be careful how you offer advice. Always leave room for your friend to disagree and reject your advice without rejecting you.

• *Learn to say you're sorry.* No one is perfect. We all make mistakes. But if you offend your friend, learn quickly to apologize and try to make it up before it becomes a stumbling block between you.

• *Learn to forgive and forget.* Your friend isn't perfect either, and will make occasional mistakes that offend you. Talk out such conflicts if you can in a calm, reasonable way. Then forgive and forget if you want to remain friends. Don't ever bring it up again.

• *Allow your friends some space.* We once knew a woman desperate for friends who would eagerly latch on to each new female arrival in the neighborhood. She would hang around her constantly and expect the newcomer to do everything with her. This usually lasted about a week, until the other woman got fed up with having no more independence and broke off the relationship. Then another new neighbor would arrive and the cycle would start all over again. It's great to have close friends, but you can't force it. Don't try to pressure people into more closeness than they're ready for. It only drives them away. Realize that your friends will want to do some things without you. That's not a rejection; it's just normal.

• *Overcome psychological barriers to interpersonal warmth.* Some people have picked up emotional scars from previous rejections. Now they find it harder to reach out and open up to others. There's no easy way around this problem, but you can work on it. Seek advice from someone you trust or even get counseling if the problem is severe. Recognize this problem in others and demonstrate boundless patience and support if you want to befriend them and help them work through such issues.

Becoming a friend isn't easy or automatic. It takes work. But the rewards far outweigh the costs. And having friends is part of what makes us human, makes us healthy, and happy, and fulfilled.

CHAPTER 46

Put Away Problems

In our search for friends and human relationships and other aspects of our daily interpersonal interactions, we sometimes come across not friendly, but unpleasant people—people more likely to disturb than delight us. Sometimes it's easier to avoid such a person once you've identified him or her. But sometimes you can't, as when you share an office with one, live next door, or work closely together in the same community organization. Then what? How best to deal with it?

To a certain degree, everyone is unique. Yet there are enough general characteristics among chronic troublemakers that we can group them into a few recognizable categories.

Basic Types of Problem People

- *Mr. Chip-on-the-Shoulder.* This guy is a hothead. He seems to look for annoyance in things others do no matter how well intentioned they are. You never know when he's going to get red in the face and explode with anger.

- *The Back Stabber.* When face to face, this person may seem pleasant. But you find out later that she did something hurtful behind your back, either spreading gossip, blabbing secrets you entrusted to her, or even lying to get you into trouble.

- *The Credit Hog.* You work on a project with someone. You do an equal or even greater share, but then hear him claiming credit for the whole shebang.

- *The Teaser.* This person continually cuts you down or insults you or mocks you in hurtful ways, but if you act wounded pretends it was all a joke. If you object, she accuses you of having no sense of humor and acts as if she is the offended party.

- *The Complainer.* This person sees only the dark cloud behind every silver lining. He seems dramatically upset over every annoyance, no matter how small, and constantly wants to burden you with vocalized thoughts about each trivial little issue.

We could go on and on listing the types of behaviors with which others drive you batty. But instead let's turn now to what you can do about it.

Master Problem Situations

Understand Others' Motives

The first step in conquering a bad situation is to understand it. Once you've cooled down, try to think rationally and analytically about what happened. Ponder the several "whys" in that painful encounter:

- *"Why me?"* Why did she attack/bother/annoy you instead of someone else?

- "*Why now?*" What's going on in this person's life that made him attack or undercut you? Is he facing severe problems of his own and just using you as a scapegoat?

- "*Why this behavior?*" Why did she resort to such childish behavior instead of more mature responses to the situation?

You may not deduce the correct answers to all these questions. And seeking to understand doesn't imply that we justify bad conduct or pretend that it's acceptable. But just thinking about such issues will provide insights and better equip you to handle the next instance of that problem behavior.

Eliminate Triggers in Your Own Behavior

The answers to the question "why me?" may provide clues to something you are doing that helps trigger the behavior. Are you being attacked or bothered simply because you appear weak, a safe target? Are you unwittingly doing something that in the other person's mind could justify his response? For instance, is it possible the Teaser starts digging at you only after you've made a wisecrack, something you meant innocently but that he misinterpreted? Think what you were doing just before any such encounter and experiment by not doing it again around this person. See if it makes a difference.

Refuse to Play the Game

You could be entirely innocent in every way and still become a target. But the person is unlikely to continue in the behavior if you refuse to deliver a psychological payoff. For instance, a hostile aggressive person may use anger as a tool to intimidate others. But if you refuse to act intimidated, she may give up using that tool on you. It helps if you analyze the situation and prepare yourself in advance with a plan of action for the next occurrence.

Friendly Assertiveness

Don't fight fire with fire. That will only worsen the conflict. Instead, learn to be more assertive, but in a friendly rather than an aggressive way, with a smile rather than a scowl.

- Assume a commanding demeanor—don't slouch, lean against the door, fold your arms, look down, or in any other way appear shy or weak. Stand square on both feet and make eye contact. But don't overdo it. Try to appear relaxed rather than ready to rumble.

- Speak softly, but clearly and firmly. In an assertive encounter, never raise your voice in anger no matter what the other person does. If he gets louder, you speak softer, forcing him to be quieter so he can hear. Softer does not imply weak or wishy-washy. Speak slowly, firmly, and very clearly, but in a dignified way rather than a shout.

- Try to appear friendly and understanding, but be unambiguous about what you want. For instance, "I'm sure you didn't mean to insult me, but I would appreciate you not spreading my secrets around. Thank you."

Turn Interpersonal Conflicts Around

You may succeed at all the above steps and get what you want, but still have a wary enemy rather than a friend. See if you can win her over completely. This may not always work, but it's usually worth a try. The best way is to do something nice for her. It can be as simple as wishing her a happy birthday or openly complimenting her during a meeting at work or at a community group. Anytime you go the extra mile like this, it signals to the other person that you don't hold grudges, that you care about her as a human being, and that you're worthy of her friendship. Even if she chooses to remain an enemy, you can walk away feeling free and clear knowing that you did your best.

Putting away such problems relieves you of a lot of excess baggage. You feel—and look—more relaxed and happy. Have you ever noticed a grim and anxious person retire from work and come back for a visit in a few months looking fresh and relaxed, appearing years younger than when he left? You don't have to retire to achieve such benefits. You can bust this sign of age, improving health as well as appearance, by mastering many of your problems now. Why wait?

PART VI

Enhance Emotional Health

We'll end this book with a final set of chapters on ways to improve psychological balance and emotional satisfaction. This is the final piece of the puzzle to maximally bust the signs of age and be younger than your years. Sometimes people can get the physical things like exercise and diet straight, can do well with behavioral stuff like good habits and relationships, and still carry around some poor attitudinal baggage. Sometimes an attitude adjustment is just the thing to provide the happy icing on the cake of your life.

We'll talk first about breaking the power of negative attitudes, then proceed with ways to build more satisfaction, meaning, and joy into every facet of your life.

CHAPTER 47

Don't Get Mad, Get Healthy

W e've read of people with uncontrolled anger who literally killed themselves decades before their time—people dying at the age of thirty-eight or forty-five who otherwise might live to sixty-five or eighty. This is serious: uncontrolled rage can kill you. It drastically jolts up your blood pressure and your heart rate. You can stroke out or have a heart attack and die on the spot. A study at Brown University Medical School found that the more hostile men were, the greater their chances of heart disease. Or you can become totally irrational and accidentally kill yourself and/or others, as in the many cases of road rage leading to highway duels to the death.

Of course, we're not talking about getting a little irritated now and then, just a little upset and snappy. We all have periods where things grate on our nerves, we get a little worked up, and we say some things we shouldn't. Rather we're talking about people who seem to carry anger around with them all day like a bag of hot coals tossed over their shoulder. They may even act proud of it, thinking constant ire gives them more power by intimidating others. They may consider it as a badge of distinction, as if they were somehow superior by "being themselves" and acting unafraid to violate social convention.

But they're doing as much damage to themselves as to others. As some say, "It's not just what you eat; it's what's eating you that counts." In other words, the thoughts and emotions that you let cling to you like an enraged cat, scratching and clawing all day at your consciousness, are the things that can destroy you in time.

Anger can not only ruin your health, but also destroy your social relationships. Who wants to live long with an irate, crabby, volcano of fury who is likely to spew forth temper and wrath without warning? Uncontrolled anger is the one emotion that can cost you everything—family, friends, career, and health.

Don't let that happen! Learn to conquer your anger before it conquers you.

Judging When Anger Is Disproportionate

Anger is a natural human emotion, and sometimes you should feel angry. Anger has its good side—namely, when it motivates us to critique and challenge unjust situations. Without a sense of righteous indignation, crimes might not get reported, aggression might not be stopped, and people might not stand up for the downtrodden. Would people be as willing to stand up for their own rights in the face of harassment, bullying, and other forms of mistreatment?

So we're not telling you to ignore anger, pretend that it doesn't exist, repress it deep within the subconscious, or any kind of irrational move like that. Instead, we're suggesting you learn to keep anger proportionate to what caused it, to channel anger toward reasonable solutions, and to release angry feelings lest the bottled up pressure explode in negative ways.

Anger has gone too far when the urge to do something irrational is overwhelming. For instance, you want to kill the other person or yourself or both. You're willing to risk life and limb to catch the driver who cut you off on the interstate. You're willing to throw away your job or marriage or other relationship. You are truly making a mountain out of a molehill.

Anger is also disproportionate when you find yourself enjoying the adrenaline "high" you get from feeling so angry. There is a kind of rush as the body prepares itself for the famous "fight or flight" response. Some people get off on such feelings and thus actively seek them, whether consciously or not.

Anger is disproportionate, too, when the emotion merely expresses itself but doesn't lead toward meaningful solutions. You enjoy talking about the cause of anger, relive the experience, and may even engage in revenge fantasies, but you're unwilling to actually do anything to improve the situation that caused the anger.

Seven Ways to Keep Anger in Check During an Encounter

If your anger is disproportionate or out of control, try these suggestions:

1. *Stop and think.* The well-known advice about counting to ten before you say something makes sense. There's nothing magic about the number ten, but it is a convenient way to buy time so you can think of an appropriate (rather than devastating) response. Whether it takes you to a count of three or thirty, it's better to keep quiet until you can think of something good.

2. *Distract yourself.* The other aspect of counting to ten is that it distracts you. That is, the act of counting—or looking out the window at clouds or noting the pattern in the tiles at your feet—tends to split your concentration from the source of anger. This lessens the anger a bit so that you can reassert some self-control.

3. *Take a deep breath.* As we saw in chapter 4 on breathing, just one or two deep, slow, and regular breaths can amazingly dispel stress and tension. By itself, this won't solve the problem. But it should lessen the grip of your emotions on your mind so that you can think more clearly.

4. *Remember something positive.* If the source of your anger is

a loved one, think not of the stupid thing she just did, but of one or more of the nice things she's done in the past. Remind yourself of your love for her and how you don't want to jeopardize everything for the momentary satisfaction of anger release. If the source of your anger is someone whom you've lost respect for, you can still think of something else good. Think of your upcoming trip to Yosemite or your outing that evening to dinner and the movies. Think of anything that helps lessen the intense negativity of the moment.

5. *Prepare yourself in advance.* Sometimes you know in advance that you're about to enter a situation likely to cause anger—for example, you must confront an insubordinate employee or an unruly child. Steel yourself in advance with thoughts that you will remain calm and patient, you will do and say the right thing. If you know you must face a serious commute home, resolve in advance not to shout or curse if someone cuts you off or yells at you.

6. *Say something to defuse the tension.* In a face-to-face encounter with tempers rising on both sides, say something to dispel the dark clouds. You might, for instance, make a light comment about the encounter itself—"Well, now, this isn't going as well as I'd hoped!" Just make sure you don't do it in an angry, aggressive, or mocking fashion, or you'll likely add to the lightning and thunder.

7. *Relax your facial muscles.* When you're tense and angry, your facial muscles become rigid and contorted. You may not be aware of it in yourself, but note the other person—he or she probably shows it. Look in the mirror and you might surprise yourself with your own expression! Each person sees such expressions on the other's face, and it's like waving a red flag before a bull. It just escalates the strife further. Tone things down by deliberately forcing your face back to a normal expression. This takes practice, but you can do it. The other person will probably relax some then, too.

Releasing Steam After an Encounter

Hopefully the above techniques will see you through to some satisfactory resolution during an angry encounter. But afterward, you still may feel as if you have steam coming out of your ears. That's due to the adrenaline-induced autonomic nervous system arousal, which doesn't simply dissipate after the problem is over, even if it ended well. The best thing now is to get exercise (see all of part I), talk it out with a close friend or loved one, or seek relaxation in a favorite pastime.

The Last Resort When Everything Else Fails

What if all other efforts at self-control let you down? Perhaps the provocation is extreme, or your control mechanisms are worn out due to fatigue and other stresses besides the anger, and you feel you're about to blow your top. There's one final trick that almost always works, but don't overuse it or you'll wear it out, rendering it less effective in the future.

Laugh! That's right, laugh. Note something silly or crazy about the situation and let your feelings all explode forth in laughter rather than anger. This can really work. Our youngest child, when she was about two years old, was sitting in her father's lap when she dropped her drink, spilling it all over the chair, the floor, and him. This was a genuine accident, not a temper tantrum. She looked at the mess, then up at her dad. Charles had had a tough day at work and was tired but he suddenly realized how inappropriate and ridiculous any anger would be in this situation. Instead he laughed, hugged her, and helped her clean up the mess. Her anxiety disappeared in a flash, and all was right with the world again.

CHAPTER 48

Learn to Cope With Frustration

When someone or something blocks you from reaching a goal, how does that make you feel? *Happy, friendly,* and *content* aren't the words that spring to mind, are they?

Five Typical Negative Responses to Frustration and Disappointment

1. *Anger.* You signal to change lanes to pass the slow guy in front of you, but some driver out of the blue zooms forward and blocks you. You become outraged and furious! Your heart pounds and your sweaty hands rigidly clench the wheel.

2. *Active aggression.* Road rage leads to countless accidents and deliberate attacks every year. Decades ago, a group of scientists at Yale postulated that frustration always leads to some form of aggression, and observed that aggression always results from frustration. They reasoned that if you can't attack the source of your frustration directly, your muted anger will emerge in some other form—perhaps a later argument with your spouse, yelling at the kids, or mistreating the poor dog.

3. *Passive aggression.* Some people don't actively attack the source of their frustration, but they get even by refusing to do things they should. Mad at his boss, the frustrated laborer slows his pace or deliberately makes costly or time-consuming mistakes. Others will spite people they're annoyed with by avoiding them, withholding favors, refusing to speak to them, and so on.

4. *Sulking.* This one isn't quite active or passive aggression, but rather an indirect sort. The frustrated person makes his or her upset feelings apparent with pouty facial expressions, sarcasm, and other verbal and nonverbal expressions of discontent. The aim is to psychologically make the other person feel guilty.

5. *Giving up.* Some people get so frustrated in their pursuit of goals that they just give up. After a few rejections, the unemployed person may quit looking for a job, perhaps resorting to alcoholism, drug abuse, or other self-destructive behaviors. In such cases, giving up becomes a form of aggression directed at the self.

Dire Consequences From Negative Reactions to Frustration

- *Heart problems.* As we saw in chapter 47, people who carry a lot of anger around with them, whether they express it openly or not, tend to develop high blood pressure and dramatically increase their risk of heart attacks and strokes. In fact, a fatal episode is often triggered by an uncontrolled outburst of anger.

- *Strife and conflict.* Continually frustrated and angry people naturally alienate others. They rupture or prevent the formation of close interpersonal relationships. Instead, they engender conflict wherever they go—often without realizing that they themselves are the primary cause!

- *Psychological distress.* Unresolved tension keeps your mind and body in a state of stress. It becomes difficult to relax, to have fun, to enjoy life. Physically and mentally, you just keep paying for your inability to control the frustration-aggression connection.

Positive Ways to Handle Frustration

You don't have to resort to the negative behaviors just described. There is a better way.

- *Realize that everyone experiences frustration.* Obviously, each person is most attuned to his or her own special problems. But when you feel that you really are the only one with frustration, or at least with such a magnitude of it, you tend to feel anger all the more at God or the whole outside world. You tend to feel sorry for yourself and wallow in self-pity. Once you realize that everyone has problems such as yours, however, you begin to gain perspective on the issue.

- *Break the frustration-aggression bond.* Just because the two are often linked doesn't mean they have to be. You're not a machine that must respond aggressively every time a frustration approaches. You're a rational human being with willpower as well as feelings. Next time you get frustrated, stop and think before you lash out emotionally. Let your logical mind take control. Emulate *Star Trek's* Mr. Spock. Act like a rational Vulcan.

- *Overcome frustrating barriers.* Once you gain control over yourself, you can start to think of ways to overcome the barricades standing between you and reaching your goal. Be creative and adaptive, not aggressive. Keep your mind fixed on the goal rather than fretting and stewing in anger at the barrier. Approach the problem from a fresh angle, think creatively, and try out any good ideas that pop into your mind. If the first one doesn't work, try another. And then another. A Thomas Edison doesn't create a breakthrough for all humanity on his first attempt to create a lightbulb. But unlike too many of us, an Edison doesn't quit. He keeps plugging away until he succeeds.

- *Change your goal when you must.* Some goals are unrealistic, and you should give up on them. There's a place for the kind of persistence exemplified by Edison—and there's also a place for realizing that you had the wrong goal in the first place. For example, if your goal is to court and marry a certain other person and all he or she does is reject your every overture, *don't* play an Edison. You're just asking for more heartbreak, and acting more like an obsessed fan than a responsible person. Give up and move on to another person who shares your interest in building a relationship.

When trying to control your reactions to frustration, it's easy to become frustrated about your own inability to perfectly do what you wish you could. In other words, you can become frustrated about your inadequate response to frustration. Then you feel tempted to give up. Try to avoid this vicious spiral. Sure, you'll make mistakes. But just keep accepting yourself as the flawed person you are and keep trying. You may never become perfect, but you'll achieve a lot more by trying and occasionally failing than by never even trying at all.

CHAPTER 49

Adopt A Pet

Human friends come and go. We move away from them, or they depart from us. Some tiff arises and grows into a major conflict that ruptures the relationship. They criticize or reject us, wounding our pride or hurting our feelings.

But animal friends tend to stay for life. We take them with us when we move. They accept us when we have a bad hair day, wake up in a foul mood, or make mistakes at work. If we've selected the right species and breed, they greet us warmly, lovingly, joyously whenever we return. For some people, it may be the highlight of the day.

We certainly don't want to discourage you from working at your human relationships. But if you want additional solace and companionship, consider getting a pet.

The Many Benefits of Pets

Scientific studies have amply demonstrated these psychological and medical benefits of loving pets. They:

- *Reduce loneliness.* Most people can't stand an empty house or apartment. If you lack human companions, try a pet.

- *Boost feelings of security.* Dogs, in particular, are great for alerting you to intruders or warning them away.

- *Enhance happiness.* Love—even that for a pet—makes you happier and more optimistic.

- *Lower blood pressure.* Simply petting a friendly animal lowers elevated blood pressure. It also relaxes you when you're tense. For instance, a study of hypertensive New York stockbrokers taking blood pressure medicine, conducted by the University of Buffalo, found that those with pets kept their blood pressure under control even when under stress, but those without pets didn't. Similarly, watching fish swim in an aquarium relaxes people and lowers their blood pressure.

- *Extend life.* Studies of the elderly in nursing homes show that having pets makes the residents healthier—and they live longer, too.

Decide If You're a Good Candidate for Pets

Pets aren't for everyone. If you don't really want one, are away from home too much, or too irresponsible to care for one properly, please, please don't get one.

Take This Quiz

We developed the following Pet Attitude Scale, originally published in *The Psychological Record* 31 (1981). Take this survey to see if you have the kind of attitudes associated with loving and caring for pets. Just answer each question *true* or *false* according to how you feel right now.

1. I really like seeing pets enjoy their food.

2. My pet means more to me than any of my friends.

3. I would like a pet in my home.

4. Having pets is a waste of money.

5. House pets add happiness to my life (or would if I had one).

6. I feel that pets should always be kept outside.

7. I spend time every day playing with my pet (or I would if I had one).

8. I have occasionally communicated with a pet and understood what it was trying to express.

9. The world would be a better place if people would stop spending so much time caring for their pets and started caring more for other human beings instead.

10. I like to feed animals out of my hand.

11. I love pets.

12. Animals belong in the wild or in zoos, but not in the home.

13. If you keep pets in the house, you can expect a lot of damage to furniture.

14. I like house pets.

15. Pets are fun, but it's not worth the trouble of owning one.

16. I frequently talk to my pet.

17. I hate animals.

18. You should treat your house pets with as much respect as you would a human member of your family.

Scoring

For each of the following you answered *true*, score one point: items 1, 2, 3, 5, 7, 8, 10, 11, 14, 16, and 18. A *false* on any of these means a zero for that item.

For each of the following answered *false*, score one point: 4, 6, 9, 12, 13, 15, and 17. Now add up your total score. If you scored 12 or less, you probably aren't a good candidate for pet ownership. If you feel you must get one anyway, consider a less personal pet like tropical fish or reptiles.

If you scored 13 through 15, consider getting a pet if you have the time and resources to care for it properly.

If you scored 16 through 18 and don't already have a pet, then go for it if you can!

Get Your Perfect Pet

To start with, follow your natural inclination. For example, some people just instinctively prefer cats, while others opt for dogs.

Once you've decided on a category, let's plan a bit more rationally. Consider the known physical and behavioral traits rather than just how cute they look in the shop window. Puppies do grow up and change, you know. And different breeds have widely disparate behaviors.

Consider such factors as ultimate size, feeding bills, activity levels, space available for play, and aggressiveness with strangers and children. Legitimate pet store owners can make realistic recommendations when informed about what you want. There are also books available that may help (consult your local bookstore or library).

Finally, if you have access to the Internet, you can visit the following sites to specify the characteristics you want and find out which breeds best meet your requirements:

- http://www.purina.personalogic.com.

- http://www.puppyfinder.com (for dogs).

- http://selectsmart.com (for many sorts of pets, from dogs or cats to horses).

Other sites may help with caring for your pet once you get it; try http://www.healthypet.com, for instance.

Having pets can be a really fun way to slow your biological clock!

CHAPTER 50

Learn to Relax

A certain amount of stress energizes you. If you were too laid back, too unconcerned, you might just let important duties, taskers, and responsibilities slip through your fingers. But there isn't much of a margin between the level of stress that energizes you and the higher levels that begin to paralyze you. At this point, panic can set in and cause such effects as these:

- *You lose all creative ability.* Just when you most need some fresh thinking to solve your problems, this capacity vanishes.

- *You get emotionally upset, angry.* You waste a lot of energy on emotions that conflict with your ability to handle the tasks at hand.

- *Your body is in turmoil.* You can feel the tension burning in your guts. It's hard to rest, or eat, or enjoy life. You feel sick inside and may actually experience pretty severe psychosomatic symptoms such as vomiting or diarrhea. (*Psychosomatic*, by the way, means that your mind really is affecting your body; it doesn't mean that something is "only in your mind.")

- *Ruptured relationships.* People see your misery and hostility and don't want to be with you.

So how do you get off this crazy tilt-a-whirl?

Break the Cycle

Distract Yourself

When you feel like a blender with a loose lid that's about to blow all its contents, push the *off* button! That's right, just *stop* once in a while. Not while you're on the interstate changing lanes, of course, but at opportune moments just take a break. If you can get up and walk away from the desk, kitchen, or other place of stress, so much the better. If not, just pause mentally from the task at hand and think. Look at that picture of your loved ones. Remind yourself what this is all about. Take a few minutes to read the paper or check the headlines on the Internet or glance at that joke memo people have been passing around. Call someone friendly on the phone and swap horror stories. Go get a drink of water or take a bathroom break. Look out the window at the beauty of the clouds or trees or whatever you can see. Even just a minute or two like this may help break that stress cycle—temporarily, at least.

Progressive Muscle Relaxation

To counteract all the effects of stress on your body and mind, however, you'll need to do a bit more along the lines of deep muscle relaxation. This takes time, so you may not be able to do it until a longer break is possible.

It helps if you can get into a comfortable position away from major sensory stimulation or other people who would interrupt you. If you're at home and can lie down, great. But you can also do this with your head on your folded arms on your desk, or even sitting upright as long as you can lean back and let yourself go.

Close your eyes, and focus on one group of muscles at a time. It's usually better to start at one end of your body and work in sequence toward the other end. For example, start with your head and work down toward your feet, or vice versa. At each point, briefly tense your muscles and then note how the tension fades as you relax them. Keep relaxing each major group in turn, while noting if any already relaxed have grown tense again. If they have, go back and relax them again. With a bit of practice, you won't have to tense your muscles first at all. You'll be able to tune in to the level of tension they already have and ramp it down several notches almost instantly.

Once you have all your muscles relaxed, start thinking pleasant thoughts—the relaxing kind, not something exciting like winning the lottery. Just visualize the most peaceful and enjoyable place you've ever been to or can imagine. Bring all your sensory capacities into play. If it's the beach, for example, imagine not only the visual scene of the waves lapping softly over the sand, but also the warmth of the sun, the sound of gulls, the smell of the fresh air, the delicious taste of cold iced tea.

The Joys of Relaxation

You may achieve a deep state of physical and mental relaxation even in your first session of ten to twenty minutes. Some people, however, need multiple sessions of practice to develop this gentle technique. But it shouldn't take long for you to gain enough control to simply erase the tension of the past few hours and replace it with blissful relaxation. Then you'll experience benefits like these:

- You'll feel rested, more able to cope.

- You'll calm those negative emotions and their draining effects on your body.

- You'll get more creative again, with super insights and ideas bursting out of your subconscious mind. Often you'll find the very answer you need, the one that kept eluding you when your mind boiled over with multiple demands.

- You'll feel younger and healthier and happier.
- You'll look younger and healthier and happier, too.

CHAPTER 51

Choose to See the Glass Half Full

Everyone has problems in life. Everyone worries about situations like these:

- *Relationships.* With parents and children, with spouses or intimate friends, with bosses or coworkers.

- *Physical appearance.* Feeling too fat or too thin, too tall or too short, some body part seeming too big or too small, or feeling unattractive for any other reason.

- *Health.* Some chronic illness, weakness, or other condition that vexes and worries you or never seems to get better.

- *Financial status.* No matter how much money you have, it never seems to be enough. Expenses and other demands always seem to catch up with or exceed income no matter how big a raise or promotion or bonus you get.

- *Possessions.* Cars, appliances, and other devices are constantly breaking down, getting lost, or requiring maintenance and replacement.

It's absolutely normal to have problems like these. We all do. We always will. The only question is, will you let such difficulties ruin your outlook on life or will you master them?

Resilience

Some people are better than others at bouncing back after life knocks them flat. Before the count of ten, they jump back on their feet and are throwing punches again. They conquer their problems and emerge victorious. Psychologists have coined the term *resilience* for this ability to sustain hardship yet never give up, but keep fighting back until you win. The resilient person looks at setbacks not as defeats but as challenges to overcome.

The good news is that however little or much resilience you now possess, you can develop more. You can strengthen this skill or approach to life. Your new, more positive attitude can help keep you happy, healthy, and successful despite whatever negative circumstances assault you.

Sybil and Steven Wolin, who run Project Resilience (a private organization in Washington, D.C., that studies people who have overcome terrible childhoods), have identified seven key aspects of resilience that you can work on, some of which we have discussed in earlier chapters but will mention again.

1. Morality

You need to have or develop a moral compass, a sense of right and wrong. Morality helps guide you in the correct direction and motivate you to keep moving toward what you know is right despite difficulties.

2. Independence

Do you remember as a kid begging for the freedom to do something that "everyone else was doing"? And what did your parents say? "If everyone else jumped in the lake, would you do it, too?" Resilient people don't follow the crowd. They think for themselves and act independently, whether anyone else supports them or not.

3. Insight

If you're willing to stand up for what's right and act independently, you'd better pray for a good measure of insight so that you don't make stupid mistakes. You don't want to dart about jousting at windmills or taking on other fruitless quests. Ask deep and probing questions, gather information, and mull it over until the answer comes to you. The correct path should become a clear vision in your mind, something you feel strongly you must do. If your vision remains muddled, keep thinking before you make up your mind or commit yourself.

4. Creativity

Creativity goes hand in hand with insight, helping you break out of your rut. It helps you remain independent as you develop plans and strategies that no one else you know has apparently thought of or tried. Your original approach may be just the one to work, helping you leap over the barrier that has left others feeling hopeless and defeated.

5. Initiative

Once you've exercised creativity and insight and come up with a plan, initiative gets you moving so that you actually implement it. Lots of people get good ideas. They may even talk a lot about their great plans and projects. But then they do nothing. To have resilience, to become a winner, means that you get out there and do something about reaching your goals.

6. Relationships

Being independent doesn't imply that you must be a loner. You need to maintain warm, open, honest, intimate relationships with others to remain happy and productive. What fun is success if you plan to remain forever alone? Close relationships help sustain you when things temporarily don't go your way. They provide incentives—if you're going to "bring home the bacon," it's nice to have someone to bring it home to.

7. Humor

Despite all your best efforts, things will sometimes go wrong. You'll be tempted to feel dejected and blue. At such times, look for the humor in the situation. Or take a break from your exertions and see a funny movie or other show. Laughter can often be the best medicine and provide the respite and stress relief you need to recharge your batteries before you again enter the fray.

Resilience is a beautiful concept. Think of trees being tossed by powerful storm winds. Some bend too much, and grow up crooked afterward. Some refuse to bend, but then snap in two when the wind grows forceful and destructive enough. Others are resilient and, though tossed to and fro for a time, bounce back into position to grow tall and straight and magnificent. The wind has not weakened or defeated them, but rather made them stronger.

CHAPTER 52

Exercise Your Faith

The late Victor Frankl, a Viennese psychiatrist, endured the horrors of Nazi concentration camps during World War II. Later he wrote a book called *Man's Search for Meaning*, and several follow-up books on the same theme. What he learned by difficult personal experience is that people in the death camps who had no sense of meaning in life commonly gave up, wilted away in the oppressive atmosphere, and died. But others, though suffering the exact same level of deprivation and maltreatment, retained a sense of meaning and emerged from the horror relatively unscathed in terms of mental health.

U.S. military prisoners of war in the Vietnam War who survived months or even years of terrible torture, ridiculously inadequate diet, lack of medical care, and psychological abuse often reported similar perceptions. Those with a sense of purpose, meaning in life, and faith in God could often survive horrible ordeals. Such people didn't merely survive in the sense of tenaciously but barely clinging to life by the skin of their teeth. Rather, they sometimes found it to be a profound growth experience in terms of their personality, maturity, interpersonal relationships, and aims in life. See, for example, Admiral Jeremiah Denton's book *When Hell Was in Session*. Denton later became an admired U.S. senator. Others with similar experiences such as John McCain are still (as of this writing) in the Senate or in other major positions of national leadership.

Most of us can scarcely imagine enduring what these particular heroes did. But all of us have problems in life. All of us at times feel mistreated, isolated, rejected, put upon. These types of difficulties are so much less than the horrors just mentioned, so why can't we also face our own predicaments more positively, with dignity and a sense of purpose?

The Bible tells us that when everything else is stripped away—our successes, our power, our possessions, all of our status, and the toys and distractions we so often rely on—only three things still remain: faith, hope, and love. These three can see you through anything else that ever besets you in life. In the quiet times, develop a solid foundation in these three areas. It will see you through the stormy days when everything else seems to go wrong. And such a foundation will actually slow your biological clock, too.

Have Faith

Innumerable scientific studies have shown that people with faith have better physical and mental health. For instance, one of Charles's studies among students at the University of Pennsylvania found that those who considered themselves atheists or agnostics were twice as likely to be in ill health as were those with faith.

Other studies have shown that people who attend church regularly, or pray, tend to have healthier hearts, to recover faster from surgery, to be happier, to live longer even when confronted with serious diseases like cancer. There was a time when doctors were trained rigorously to trust only the scientific approach to medicine, and to discount the very notion of miracles and healing through spiritual means. But when confronted with all the recent research evidence, even those physicians who themselves disbelieve in God are increasingly likely to comprehend the value of their patients' faith in the healing process. Such doctors may believe that it is only a placebo effect—which means that the phenomenon only works because of their patients' beliefs—yet still encourage this approach because of its demonstrated beneficial effects. A comprehensive analysis of two hundred earlier studies on religion and health conducted by Dr. Jeffrey Levin, then of the Eastern Virginia Medical School, found a strong overall association between religious faith and good health. Data like these tend to convince even the most skeptical of physicians.

Hope

Faith doesn't only give people the perception that even their suffering has some value in the divine plan for their lives. It also helps by giving them hope that things will be okay, will turn out all right in the end. As the saying goes, there are no atheists in foxholes. Most people who are in dire circumstances reach out, cry to God for help, even if they've never before had a sense of knowing or trusting Him at all. How much better to fully integrate faith throughout all phases of life. Then when you need help, you'll have more hope that it's really there and not merely some illusion. Having hope keeps you more optimistic about life, more able to see the light at the end of the tunnel than just the darkness and sharp rocks within it.

Love

This is the third and greatest of those foundational values that give meaning and joy to life. And all three go together. Without faith and hope, it's difficult to love in the deepest, truest sense. We don't mean here love as mere affection or attraction or romance as seen in the movies. We are talking about that deepest and most wonderful type of love that draws people together in mutual devotion, respect, and caring for life, no matter what happens.

Faith tells you that all of your life dilemmas have purpose and give meaning. Hope tells you that things will turn out all right in the end. Together they set you free to love when circumstances turn grim, when things are turned inside out and upside down and it seems that no power on earth can set them right. No power on earth can. But God's love can. Tuning into God's love gives you the confidence to have faith and hope.

The three—faith, hope, and love—go together as package. You are a lot better off if you accept, and seek, and grow in all three.

Index